# Don't Get a SMALL Bang For Your BUCK

# Don't Get a SMALL Bang For Your BUCK

## Think Like a Doctor; Act Like a Patient

Dr. Walter O Ochan

ISBN-13: 9781975614775
ISBN-10: 1975614771
Library of Congress Control Number: 2017913218
CreateSpace Independent Publishing Platform
North Charleston, South Carolina

# Table of Contents

# Acknowledgments

A book without a reader is no book. Thank you for buying or borrowing this book.

The core of this book came from my family unit, the people I encounter daily, and the Almighty. A family unit is almost nonexistent without a wife and mother—thank you, Lucia O. Children form the larger part of the nucleus in our family; the background noise from Andiswa, Siyabonga Latim, Siyanda Lagen, and Aphiye made writing a pleasurable process. Ayoo, a random second hand book you bought for me helped sharpen my pen. Gogo C S Sibiya, thanks for giving me three extra "wives", being the regular visiting "doctor" and being the ever present "big mother" in our lives.

Thank you, Auntie Betty, Patro, and Uncle Richard (may your soul rest in peace), for taking over where my late mum and dad stopped. Toto, Mwena, and Wac-ma-tino (may your souls rest in peace), it is a pity I never got to share my adult life with you. My large family of "the girls," "the boys," and the "three mothers" all made it nice being a son of Obal.

I would also like to acknowledge the roles played by my schools (Bungatira Central, Kiswa, *LaysCo*/Layibi College, and *N'ngo*/ Namilyango College) and my three *big schools* (Makerere University,

University of Pretoria, and University of Cape Town). A portion of this book came from each of these three varsities. Profs. S. Luboga, Kagimu, Katabira, Kakande, and all senior colleagues from MUK, you all laid a good foundation. Teachings of the late Prof. W. Wamukota formed some of the writing in this book; may your soul rest in peace. Thanks to Ann Mathews, Dr. L. Nkombua, and Dr. Liz Gwyther for the writing skills. Bungatira, my village, produced the raw boy whom the schools refined.

Portia, Niel, and Eugene, thanks for the graphics. The inspiration of the spiritual leaders at COTH International is of immense value. This book is also dedicated to Room Q24 @ Afro-Stone and the *Orphans* of Makerere University (1986–1992); medical school was fun because of the *Orphanage of MUK*. "Pastor" John Nkusi (Dr.), you have been an inspiration when it comes to *gathering* postgraduate papers from the big schools.

These books, authors, and editors (among many others) have been "manufacturing" doctors for years, and they crafted me, among others, into a doctor:

- J. F. Munro and I. Campbell, *Macleod's Clinical Examination*, 10th ed.
- I. R. McWhinney, *A Textbook of Family Medicine*.
- M. Longmore, I. B. Wilkinson, and S. Rajagopalan, *Oxford Handbook of Clinical Medicine*.
- R. B. Taylor, *Manual of Family Practice*, 2nd ed.
- M. Swash and S. Mason, *Hutchinson's Clinical Methods*.
- B. Mash, *Handbook of Family Medicine*.
- M. Watson, C. Lucas, A. Hoy, and J. Wells, *Oxford Handbook of Palliative Care*, 2nd ed.

- J. Cassidy, D. Basset, R. J. Spence, and M. Payne, *Oxford Handbook of Oncology*, 3rd ed.
- N. A. Boon, N. R. Colledge, B. R. Walker, and J. A. A. Hunter, *Davidson's Principles and Practice of Medicine*, 20th ed.
- B. Mash and J. Blitz-Lindique, *South African Family Practice Manual*, 2nd ed.
- J. Murtagh, *General Practice*, 4th ed.

In this text, material taken from these books has been digested and made easy to read and ready for absorption by nonmedical readers. Enjoy the absorption.

Dr. W. O. Ochan

# Introduction

## Buying and Selling Health

Have you ever walked out of a medical consultation and felt that you got very little in return for your coin? Someone who walks into a convenience store with a dollar would usually come out with goodies worth a dollar, compared to one who sometimes takes a dollar to the doc and walks out with ten cents' worth of health. The doctor does not do that on purpose; you just do not know how to get the most out of your dollar. This book will help you get a bigger bang for your health buck every time you visit a doctor.

Before your next medical consultation, get to think like a doctor. To think like a doc, you should get to know a bit about

- the *art* of medicine;
- the *science* of medicine;
- the *business* of medicine; and
- the *politics* of medicine.

Thinking like a doctor will not make you lose the *privilege* of being a patient; instead it will let you get the benefits of both sides of the stethoscope. You become better at giving your story to doc. This book will help you acquire the basic skills of thinking about your medical consultation and symptoms like a doctor. The book won't turn you into a doctor after a few pages. Rather, it is about helping you present your *case* to your doctor like a doc would present a *medical case* to other doctors for their expert opinions. It is like having a private doc that you carry around, and who talks to other doctors on your behalf.

In medical training (and practice), a junior doctor learns from senior medics by

- being given a medical challenge in the form of a patient;
- listening to the patient's medical story, which contains the symptoms;
- asking the patient some more questions to get at other hidden stories;
- physically examining the patient, looking for clinical signs (evidence) that may (or may not) be in agreement with the patient's story;
- running medical tests to confirm or rule out the suspected disease; and
- coming up with a management plan for the medical challenge.

The young doc then puts together the story (symptoms), evidence (signs), and test results, and the sum total is the diagnosis, which he or she presents—like a lawyer presenting a legal case to a judge—to a senior doctor. The senior doc then hears the whole story about the patient as told by the junior doc. This is the *medical case presentation.*

This is what your doctor has gone through over many years in order to become a fine doc. By the way, you can always warn your doc not to call you a "case." You are human first and then a patient, not a case!

At the end of the case presentation, the senior doc wants to know what the likely diagnosis is and what the other possible diagnoses could be—given the symptoms, signs, and the results of the basic tests. The senior doc will then want to know what the best line of management of the disease will be, and what needs to happen if the chosen management plan does not work. The junior medic is also quizzed about the possible complications of the treatment chosen.

## The Arithmetic of Medical Consultation

Your doctor's medical training gives him or her the ability to deduce what is going on inside you without *getting inside* you. This may be based on your medical story only, or on your story and physical examination. Sometimes the doc has no diagnosis till some tests are done, a second opinion is sought, or the clock has ticked on. At times we only get a diagnosis at postmortem, but fortunately, with advances in medicine, this is becoming less frequent.

(Your Story) + (Physical Examination) + (Medical Tests) + (Referrals) + (Passage of Time) = (The Diagnosis and Management of Your Health Problems)

Note: the diagnosis does not always have to have a *fancy* disease label attached to it.

After reading this book, you will walk into a doctor's room not as a case but as a patient who knows his or her own case presentation. Most times you may not know your diagnosis. Not knowing your diagnosis when you consult is not a problem; the problem is not being able to tell your whole story. Your diagnosis will not come out without a well-told story.

This book aims to help you get the most out of every medical consultation. Whether or not you have a medical problem, it is a book worth reading to help prepare you for any encounter with a medic. Eventually most of us will have to see a doctor anyway; even doctors get to consult other docs. Whether you use a private or a public health facility, a health dollar will have to be spent on your health.

When you take your health dollars to a doctor, how much health do you bring back home with you? Are you getting the best bang for your buck? Or are you getting a small bang for your buck? This is something you can change by getting more informed about the importance of your role in a medical consultation.

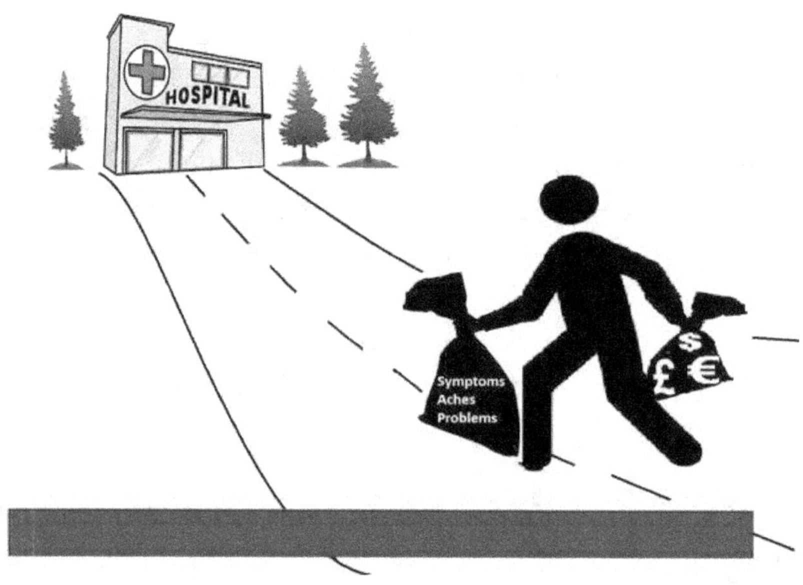


The patient depicted above should leave both parcels at the doctor's rooms and go home with a big parcel of health, but many patients leave the money bag with the doc and take the bag of symptoms back home. This book should help you leave your problems with the doc and get a bigger bang for your coin.

# One

## THIS TIME I'LL TELL THE DOCTOR EVERYTHING

### The Art of Medicine

How you tell your story to the doc is an *art* that you may need to be schooled in. Once you learn the art of telling your medical story, you will have all doctors eating out of your hand, not your pocket. The way you tell your story of pain and suffering should help your doc to make a diagnosis much faster and more cheaply. The *science* of medicine falls into place easily once you have grasped the *art* of medicine, and most of your dollar remains in your pocket. Then the *business of medicine* shall work in your favor.

You often have a specific picture that you hope to paint for the doctor; a specific health story you want to tell doc, but do not have the right story line. Your medical story is usually clear or rehearsed, but you have no clue how to give all that info effectively in just ten minutes. Some patients manage to give all the necessary info to the doctor during the short consultation time, but is that info delivered effectively or not? You need to learn the skill of delivering a powerful case presentation to your doctor.

At the beginning of the consultation, the show is yours, and you are allowed to speak your language (simple descriptions), not *doctor language*. So when the doctor gives you an opportunity to paint your medical picture, do not be at a loss.

When the doc asks, "So, Mr. Smith, how can I help you today?" you should able to take charge of the consultation. You should not panic about what to tell the doc first, and last. This art is explained more in the "Your Story" portion in the next page and beyond this chapter.

## The Business of Medicine

The medical consultation is based on

- telling the doc your story;
- the doc physically examining you, looking for *footprints* of the disease;
- you getting to endure some *medically induced pain and discomfort* in the name of medical tests;

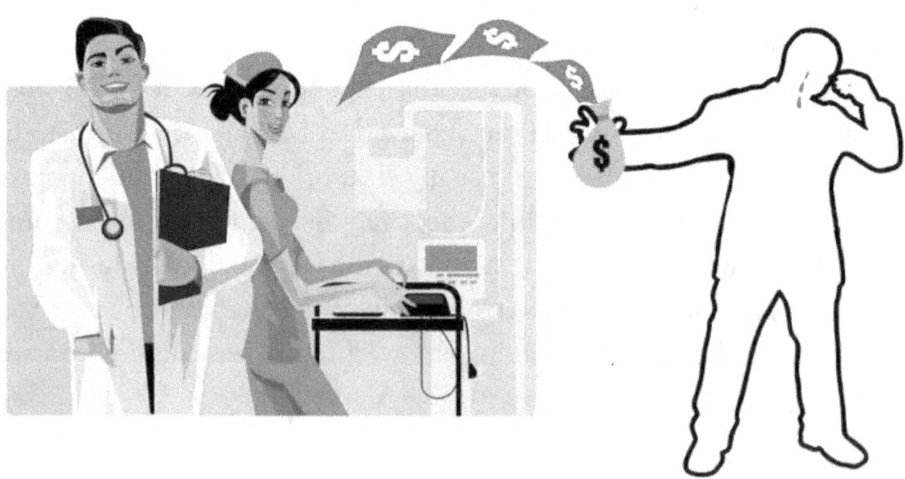

- the doc giving you *air supply* (a small pill or nothing physical to take home) and/or referral for other inputs or opinions; and
- a strategy about what should be done if the consultation does not help you as planned.
- you parting with a coin (or two) for some, or all of the above.

You may pay for all the above but you only get some of them if your story is not delivered well. Understand the art of medicine, and you benefit out of every coin you spend.


## Medical History (Your Story)

This is not about the history of medicine; it is the story of your pain and suffering. Sometimes it is called the medical interview. We may call it *story time*.

Your story time is divided into the following:

- The *big story* is your biggest symptom. It is the reason that makes you leave home, and prompts you to part with a coin.
- The *story about the big story*. You get to talk about the big story (main symptom) till you run short of words, and the doc also asks much more about this main symptom.
- The other *minor medical stories* that accompany the big story. This looks at other important medical issues that you have had but did not push you to consult. Doc does not ask a lot about these other minor symptoms.
- The *usual suspects* or the *permanent residents*: all the old medical problems that always stick around with you at all times. New illnesses come and go; the permanent residents stay put.
- Your *crowd*—that is, your family, the people around you, and those you encounter outside the home or workplace.

- What earns you a dollar every month—your job or lack of one. The things that rob you of your dollar are important and can heal you or harm you.
- The things that bring you pleasure or pain.
- Your ethnicity, belief system, and monetary health, or lack thereof.

The doc may sound like he or she wants to stereotype you by asking about all these things, but he or she actually wants to bring you (back) to health. All these things help us at diagnosis time. The "Story Time" is explained in greater details in a later chapter.

## Professional "Invasion" (Physical Examination)

Although mentioned here lightheartedly, this is a very serious medico legal issue. This part of a medical consultation has landed doctors in courts and even jails. It should be noted that physical examination invades your privacy, with your explicit permission. Doctors offer chaperones, or you could be accompanied by a friend, or family member to play chaperone. If you do not want a chaperone, most doctors may put that in writing.

This involves examination of your body, emotions, and mind. Your feelings and thoughts are assessed continually from the moment you enter the consulting room until you exit. The examination begins before you even talk.

A good history and a well-performed physical examination can save you unnecessary medical tests. Dollar bills are spent on medical tests if the history and physical examination are not done properly.

## Investigations (Medically Induced Pain)

Medical tests are a real cause of pain inflicted by doctors. The pain is felt in the pocket, in the flesh, or both. This turns doctors into socially accepted (tolerated) inflictors of pain; of course none of these are done on purpose. Blood samples are usually required to complete medical consultations. We cause you some pain in order to relieve the pain that brought you to us.


## Referrals and Retrieval

Health records from previous doctors may need to be retrieved. Sometimes referrals and consultations with other health-care workers may need to be arranged. Some medical problems require multiple specialties, hence the need to refer you to some other health-care providers. Confidential medical info about you changes hands during these exchanges.

Your consent permits these exchanges.

We have no business in sharing your medical data with doctors not involved in your health care. Third parties only get your health records with your written consent.


## Management Plans/Treatments

This is pill time, or is it? Air supply may also be the treatment of choice: you walk home with no pills but with great health. Sometimes the medical advice you get is all you need, and it is better than a packet of pills.

# Two

## The Medical Consultation

Family medicine describes a consultation as a meeting of two experts: you and your doctor. You are the expert in your symptom burden. Do not leave your doctor to guess

- how you feel;
- what you fear about your symptoms;
- why the symptoms have made you come today, and not last month or next week;
- what worries you the most about this new symptom, or recent changes in an old symptom;
- what you hope would be achieved after the consultation; or
- what you expect from this consultation.

The doctor can never pick up these things with the stethoscope. Take the guesswork out of the consultation by clarifying the main reason for consulting.

The doctor is the other expert who deduces the likely diagnosis based on your story, physical examination, medical tests, and previous health records.

Doctors of yesteryears had a saying that *the diagnosis comes from your mouth*, not the doctor's. It is still true today. When you tell your medical story in an orderly manner, the diagnosis comes out of your mouth before doc even touches you.

Give the doc your main reason for the consultation soon after the greetings and intro. You get a great consultation when you and your doctor spend much time on the main symptom.

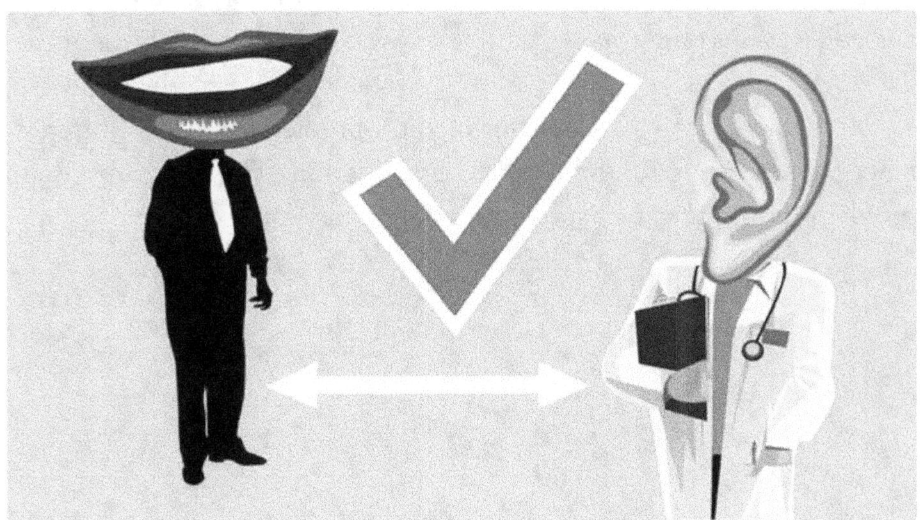

The doctor plays the big ear, and the patient is the big mouth. This demonstrates the beginning of a good consultation. Such a consultation will end up with two winners at the end.

If you realize your symptoms are arranged the wrong way around, then inform the doc, "Actually the left big toe is not the main problem, but the fire in my pants is the main problem today." The fire in the pants then becomes problem number one, and automatically the big toe becomes the least important symptom of the day and discussed last. That big toe story might as well be postponed to another day.

Knowing how to arrange your medical problems in order of importance is the key to a good medical consultation. The most important problem should top the list of your complaints to the doctor.

# Three

<br>

## STORY TIME

### The Art of Storytelling in Medicine

Indeed, you are the expert in your symptoms; you have walked around with that pain for months/years. Who else could understand your pain and suffering better than you? You may not know what the symptoms imply, but you know what they feel like and what they mean to you.

Like an artist, you should tell your story briefly but colorfully, so that the doc can feel your pain or suffering. To get healing, you need to let the doc into your world of pain or suffering. Tell your pain story well, and you shall have given doc a helping hand.

Always look at your medical symptoms as the legendary ducks: they are best lined up in a row. Make sure that the most important duck (symptom) comes first. Do not feel pity for your very tiny duckling (the least nagging symptom), and push it right to the front. The duck that quacks the loudest and nags you the most goes to the front; this is the symptom that made you consult.

Sometimes the loudest duck is not a symptom; it may be a life problem. "Doc, my wife is leaving me for my neighbor" can also be a reason for consulting. This is not a medical symptom, but it may be the loudest duck of the day. It is as good as consulting for a chest pain of sudden onset. This wife-neighbor story should be the duck that is first in the row, and the other "ducks" then follow: "Since then, I cannot sleep, eat, or concentrate at work." The duck that comes first easily explains the other ducks that follow.

Or it may be, "Doc, my husband is seeing my best friend behind my back. Ever since then, my heart is pounding out of my chest, there is a lump in my throat, I cannot eat, and neither can I sleep."

In both cases, the first problem put forward is the husband/wife issue, followed by the symptoms, and both opening remarks make for a good consultation. Both patients are likely to walk out more satisfied than another who first complains of the loss of sleep and only mentions the husband/wife problem when being issued a prescription for sleep medication at the end of the consultation. Both patients have genuine medical symptoms with social triggers.

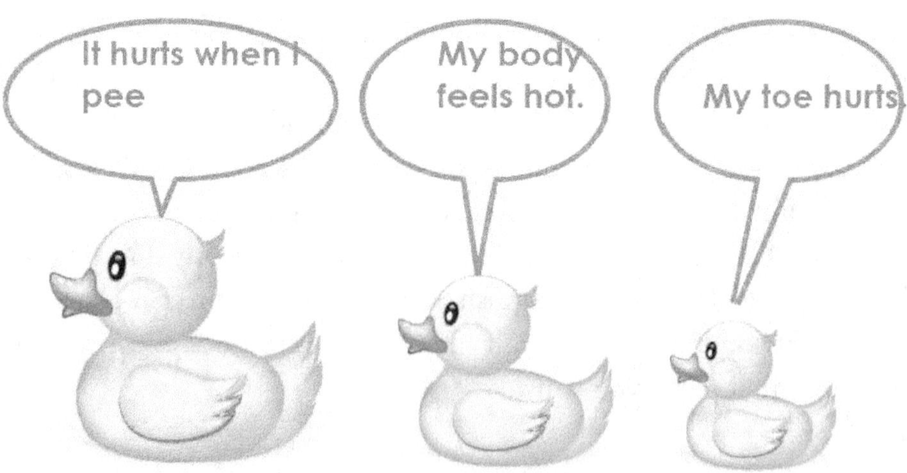

A patient who does not waste time and money is one who has severe pain when passing urine! Pain when peeing is what made him or her leave home with a health dollar. The painful pee is the first duck in the row; the painful toe is a two-year-old problem and is mentioned last (the smallest duck). Indeed, the big toe may be the first duck in the row for a patient with gout who has a sudden flare-up.

The symptom that has lasted the longest may not be your most important symptom for the day. It may have become part of your anatomy, but it can afford to wait and be mentioned as the third or fourth problem.

## The Main Story/The Biggest Symptom

The points made above guide you on how best to present your most pressing problem to your doctor. The most pressing issue or symptom is the main story. Whether it is a symptom or a socioeconomic problem, the main story should be

- the most disruptive symptom or problem;
- the most irritating symptom;
- the most alarming symptom;
- the most painful symptom;
- the most threatening symptom;
- a symptom/problem for which it is worth parting with your dollar; or
- a symptom that cannot wait for tomorrow, next week, or month.

Symptoms or problems that should also be mentioned first are those that may

- lead to loss of life if not immediately dealt with;
- signal potential damage if the symptom is not urgently addressed;

- disturb bodily function like sleep, appetite, vision, balance, and hearing;
- threaten loss of relationship and connectedness to other people;
- threaten loss of income or employability;
- threaten the loss of sanity; or
- threaten your security.

If that symptom may eventually lead to a loss of any kind, it usually should be reported first. Should you suffer any of the above losses then your doc is not to blame if you did not state your case effectively. Some of my elderly patients normally come with a handwritten list of problems (*shopping list*), and on top is usually the big-ticket symptom, the biggest medical story of the day. I guess they learnt after many years of wasted health dollars.

For you to get a good deal out of the business of medicine, you should have the full attention of your doctor. You should not just have a doctor sitting opposite you, but one whose attention is mainly focused on you. Their focus should not even be on your medical file; your file does not pay the bill.

Some good tricks of getting your doctor's full attention are given here:

- Do not start delivering the main problem before doc looks straight at you and asks, "How can I help you today?" or "What can I do for you today?"
- Do not utter the main problem if the doc is rummaging through the desk drawer without looking at you; let him or her finish, and wait till he or she invites you to talk.
- If by the time you enter the consultation room, the doctor is still looking through the previous patient's file, keep quiet even if you

have been asked to state your problem. When the doc pushes the other file aside, then you know he or she is ready for you.

- Do not state your main problem if the doc is still looking through your old medical notes and is not looking at you. After all, the new story (symptom) you have to tell may not be in your medical records. It is good to give the doc that extra minute to go through your old story in the medical file, but don't talk while the doc is focusing on your file.

- If the doc answers the phone or is called out of the consultation while you were in the middle of stating your case, start all over when the doc's attention is back on you. It is your dollar, and it is your story. If it is interrupted by that phone call, it is your duty to rephrase the story.

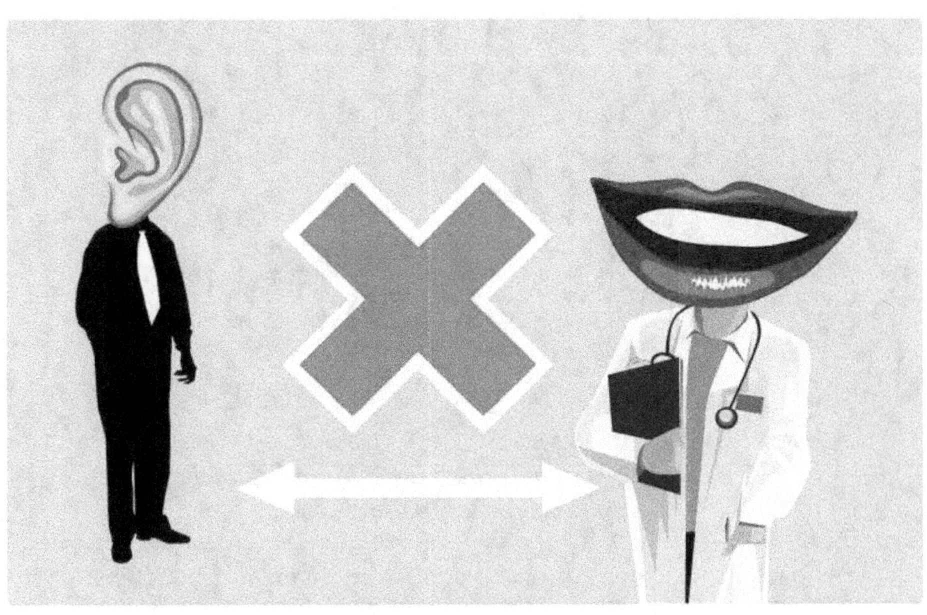

**Do not accept this "picture" at the very beginning of the consultation, it is okay only much later. Initially you should be the big mouth and doc the big ear.**

Remember that you are the storyteller, and the doctor is the listener. Doc becomes the big mouth later in the consultation. So give doc your story, starting with the most interesting part.

Sometimes the biggest symptom is accompanied by symptoms that should not be seen as separate symptoms. For example, nausea, vomiting, abdominal pain, and diarrhea can all be depicted as one duck since they are closely related. Such symptoms can all be mentioned together in one sentence; for if you leave one symptom out, you shall have interrupted the flow of your medical story. Many symptoms may also be mentioned together in the first sentence when the symptoms develop in a sequence, as if following a roster. In this scenario, the doc will allow you to tell you story the way it evolved with little interference.

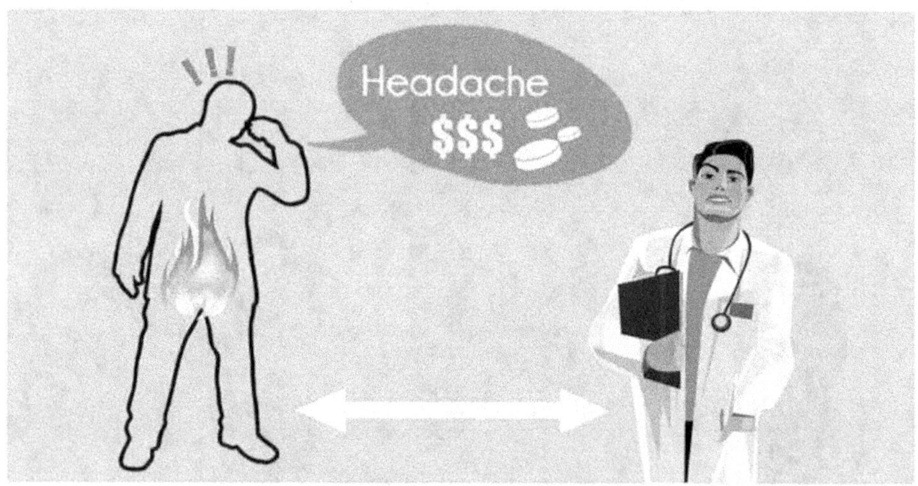



**The main problem is the "fire," but a headache story comes out. A dollar is lost.**

This patient has "fire" in one place and delivers a headache story to the doc.

The patient depicted above walks home with "fire in his pants" and a bag of headache pills that he does not need. Dollar gone for no health in return.

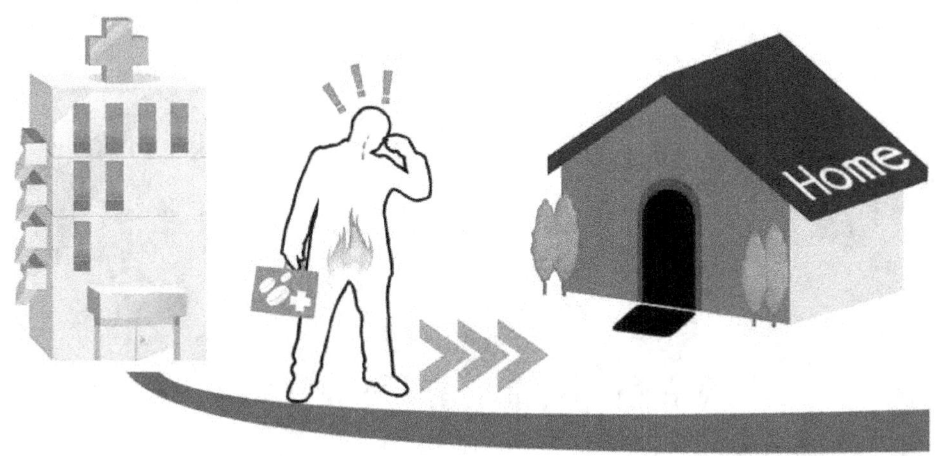


**The real problem (the fire) goes home unresolved.**

Your doctor reads you well when you state the main symptom in plain language. You will indeed impress the heck out of your doctor by avoiding fancy medical words. If you tell your story using doctor language, the doc may get lost in your symptom description. Give doc a simple story using day-to-day words. This makes you a winner; the doc quickly gets to know why you are there. Dollar saved.

# Four

## Why Do We Visit Doctors?

For one reason, or the other, most of us shall visit a doctor in our lifetime. Even doctors visit other docs. While in the waiting room, we are not one homogenous group. Each one has a specific agenda. All of us have various reasons for consulting doctors, and these include the following:

1. Administrative reasons.
If you have come purely for two days' sick leave, be frank about it. "Doc, I feel that a couple of days at home might just sort out my chest pain." You do not need to pay for x-rays for this kind of chest pain. Your doc may also become your advocate and give your employer an explanation why you could not report to work rather than a sick note.

Sometimes you just want to know if there is a connection between your work and the symptoms. If you make this clear at the onset, you save yourself and your doctor much time, unnecessary tests, and a dollar.

Some visits are for completion of medical forms. If there are no current symptoms, just present the forms and get it over and done with, and costs do not escalate.

2. Preventive reasons.

The reason is usually clear-cut; you might want a vaccine for specific reasons, routine health care, or family planning (planned parenthood). This kind of consultation is usually straightforward and not a time waster. Brief consultations usually work out cheaper, a win-win for patient and doctor. If you do not have any problem that day, just get straight to the point that brings you in. You save a dollar or two.

3. You can no longer tolerate the anxiety caused by your symptoms.

It helps to state clearly what has caused your anxiety, your *largest* and *loudest* duck. When you cannot tolerate the pain, discomfort, and other symptoms anymore, seek relief. If pain is the main symptom, then it usually has become unbearable: "Doc, I cannot stand this pain for another day." That stubborn pain is your duck number one.

4. You are failing to cope with problems of daily living.

You do not run to doc knowing that you have failed to cope; it is not that simple. When we fail to cope with the problems of daily living, our bodies help us by producing symptoms. We do not develop the symptoms knowingly; it just happens automatically. For example, we go for a consultation because we

- are failing to fall asleep or failing to stay asleep for long enough;
- are waking up unrefreshed after a full night's sleep;
- are experiencing generalized body pains not accounted for by any other medical problem; or
- are suffering from daily headaches for which all tests have proved negative.

Sometimes, after a consultation, you may see that the doctor has not grasped the reason for your visit. This is your time to clarify your story line. If you see that the doctor has arranged your ducks the wrong way around, then point out which of them is the most important.


## The Main Story/Biggest Symptom

If you feel that the pain in your tummy could be due to gallstones, you may use a simple story line: "Doc, there is this pain around my belly button, and it comes every ten to twenty minutes. I feel relieved in between these severe episodes. I vomit some dark-green stuff, and I did not sleep a wink last night. I fear it may be *my* gallstones." Here you gave a simple story about a big surgical emergency, and your doctor sets out on the right diagnostic pathway with speed and accuracy.

Without dwelling too much on the gallstone story, you shall have given your doctor vital clues about likely small bowel (intestinal) obstruction. Your gallstones are a potential source of another surgical emergency, but in this case, they are just innocent *suspects*.

The duck illustrated here shows the work of a serious patient: what took him to the doctor is breathlessness, and it is item number one (the only duck in the pond). There are no other ducks to crowd the pond. This single symptom (*duck number one*) grabs doc's attention. You do not want a pond crowded with too many ducks quacking at the same time or too many symptoms at the beginning of the consultation. Do not rely on the doctor's experience to help identify your main problem for you. You know what made you go to the doctor.

If you got a good doctor, you will note during this first part that:

- The doc keeps mum and listens/observes intently.
- The doc says nothing for the first minute, or two. This feels like a week for some patients. Don't panic; this is your time to talk and for doc to listen and not just hear you out.

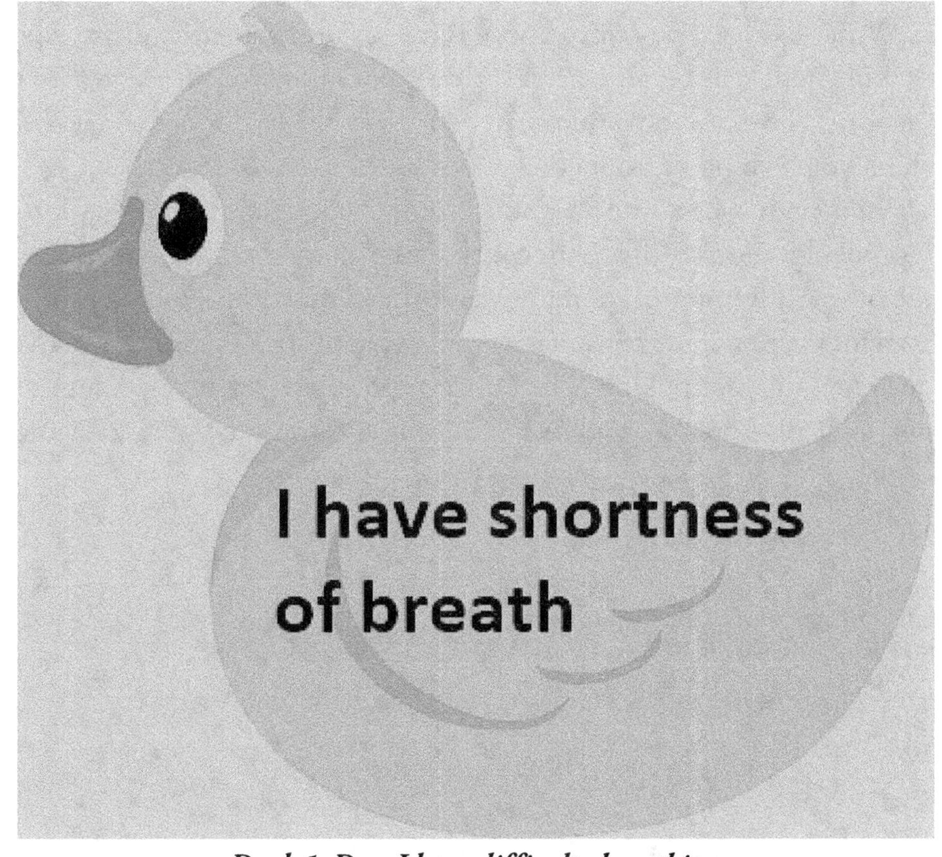


***Duck 1: Doc, I have difficulty breathing.***

- The doctor seems not to fire off any questions yet.
- You are given the liberty to describe the biggest symptom your way.
- The *big-mouth-and-big-ear* scenario plays out well here. You mentioned and described your main symptom fully; your doc listened up and listened good.

You shall not have rushed to the second or third symptom, knowing that their turns to be told would come.

What has been described above is the art of medicine: the doc zips his lips and listens because he or she does not know your story, yet. You "educate" the doc about your story, your way. The doc listens and learns about your symptom from you.

In the next phase, the doc takes over the talking, questioning, probing, poking, and also directs the course of the interview. The doc becomes the big mouth from this point onward. If you missed the above chance, then for the rest of the consultation, you will only talk in response to the doc's probing and poking. The only exception are when you want the doc to clarify some *technical words* during the consultation and at the very end, when you are given time to ask questions.

# Five

## A Detailed Look at the Big Story (History of the Main Complaint)

### The Science of Medicine

In the previous chapters, you did the storytelling your way. From here onward, you still carry on telling your story, but doc starts interjecting. The doc does not "steal" your story but starts directing you to tell the story in a way that *smells* of science. This part of storytelling works more like a *spin-doctor* for the first duck; it spends time talking about the first duck, your main symptom.

The "story about the main problem" starts discussing the main symptom in a *scientific* way. Your doc introduces a method to the storytelling. This chapter deals with four major issues, whereby the doctor

- keeps quiet and allows you to carry on;
- asks you, "Tell me more about this symptom/problem";
- takes over by asking you targeted questions about the main problem or symptom (question time begins once you have "rested

your case" and you have nothing more to say about your main symptom); and

- allows you to "rearrange your ducks" if you listed them wrongly.

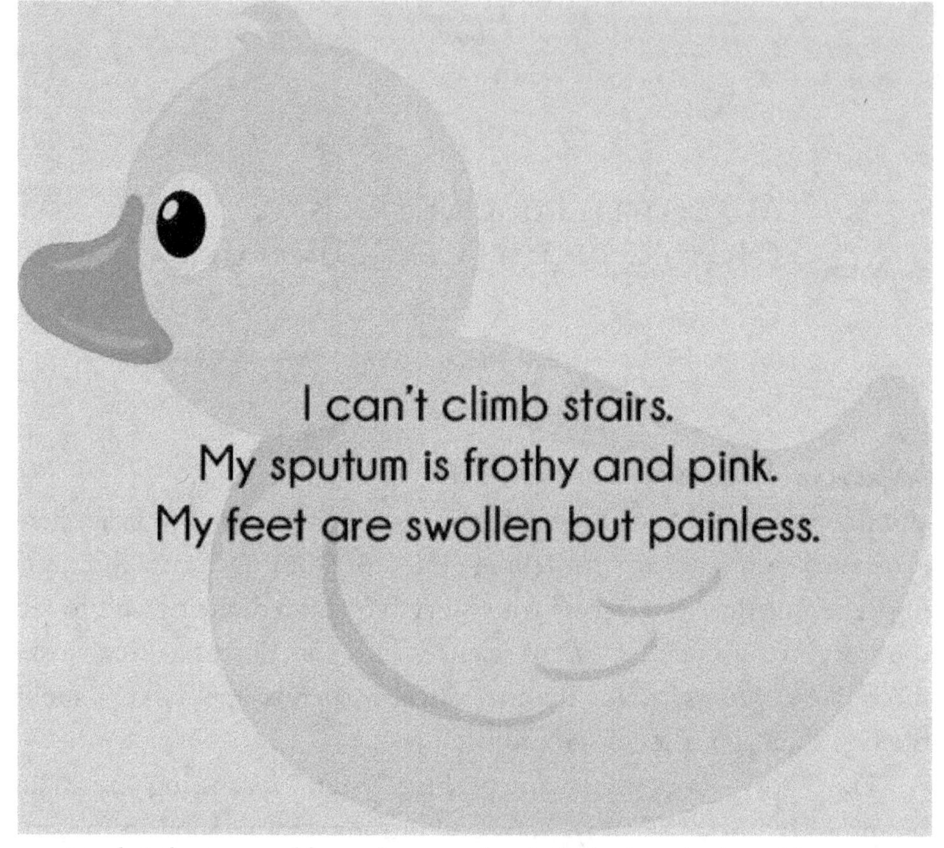


*Duck 2 depicts problems that are closely linked to the breathlessness. This describes issues that intimately go with the main symptom.*

This chapter may feel like a replay of the previous chapters, but it is the beginning of the *hunt for a diagnostic label.*

The story about the main symptom helps the doc to analyze your primary problem in great detail. A correctly stated main problem is the cornerstone of a good consultation.

## The Doc Remains Silent
### *(Your time to talk till you have nothing more to say)*

You shall have mentioned the biggest symptom earlier. At this moment talk about that main symptom, and do not list all the other problems that you may have. Describe the main problem well before mentioning other issues.

Your medical story should be like a painting meant for, or painted by, a child. A child, the small artist, would use bold but simple colors to tell a story.

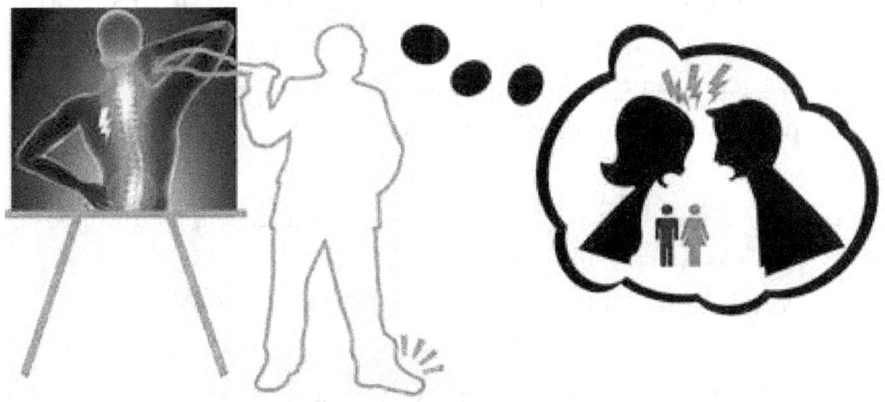

The story that brought this patient to the doctor is the constant fights with his spouse in front of their kids. The picture he is painting is of "that pain in the neck" and the old "foot story." Wrong story. Wasted paint, wasted dollar.

For your medical story to have an impact, speak *patient language*:

"My feet feel like there are ants crawling all over."
"Every time I breathe in, I feel a prick in the right side of my chest, Doc."
"Doc, my heart beats like it is about to stop, and sometimes it beats like it is about to jump right out of my chest."
"Doc, I feel like there is a frog in my throat."

The essence of patient language is simplicity.

These stories are simple descriptions that help doc to arrive at a diagnosis efficiently. Costly tests avoided, and a dollar saved.

Compared to the stories above, the following patients try to speak doctor language and usually end up complicating a consultation:

"Doc, I have acute pain in my feet."

"Doc, there is a chronic pain in my chest."

"Doc, I think I have a heart attack because I've got this heart pain."

"Doc, I have some chest complications."

"I have chronic throat inflammation, Doc."

The last one reminds me of a patient: "Doc, I have this chronic cough, but I cannot bring out the scrotum." He was thinking "sputum." By chronic cough he had meant a "bad cough." He had tried to do the *doctor talk*. To your doc, "chronic" means a symptom has lasted more than three or six months, and it may not even be severe.

When the doc remains silent, go for it. Question time will come later.

If the main symptom is shortness of the breath, then tell doc your story:

"At the beginning, I could not run to catch the bus, but I didn't worry."

"Later, I couldn't walk upstairs without resting."

"I panicked when I could not lie flat."

"There is some tightness in my chest, which worries me."

"I feel like I have gained a few pounds lately."

"These days I pass about two liters of urine at night."

Your story included issues that seem unrelated, but with that you have given the doctor your diagnosis. The diagnosis would have come out of your mouth, as they say. This has been a good *big-ear-big-mouth* moment. You did not rush to report other symptoms that you might have had for years, but elaborated a lot on the most serious and recent symptom of breathlessness. This consultation saves time for both parties. Physical examination will be focused on the problem organ or organ system, and medical tests in this case shall be specific and targeted. Dollar saved.

### *"Tell me more about that pain," says the doc*
When asked to tell the doc more, take this opportunity to talk about:

- What makes you anxious about your main problem. This is the time to say why that problem made you leave home today. If your dad died after complaining of chest pain, tell the doc, especially if your main problem is chest pain.
- Your concerns about that problem: "Doc, I'm concerned that other doctors have not taken my pain seriously."
- Your worries about the main problem: "Doc, I am worried that this pain might also take me away from my kids, like it took my dad away from us."
- Your hopes and/or expectations: "I hope that you will do some tests on my heart, but I expect that no heart problem will be discovered."
- Your fears: "I am afraid that you might also not take me seriously, like the other docs." Or: "I am afraid it is going to kill me."
- Any changes or loss in role function: "Because of the chest pain, Doc, now I cannot perform well at work or at playtime with my

kids, and my wife/husband says I have become very negative lately."

- What worsens the symptom and what makes it better: "The pain disappears when I am busy at work but gets more serious when I retire to bed at night."
- If there is a rhythm to your symptom: a particular time of day, specific events, activities, or places that provoke the symptom.
- Where it is located in the body.
- Whether it moves from one spot to another in the body or if it provokes another symptom in a different part of the body at the same time.
- Tell your story the way you would tell it to a friend: "It burns," or "It feels like ice." This gives your doctor an idea about the quality of the pain.
- If there are other unique symptoms that accompany the main problem like nausea, sweating, faintness, abnormal skin color, sudden onset of weakness, and pain in the jaw that occur together with chest discomfort. These symptoms may sound unrelated but could all point to a heart attack in a forty-year-old diabetic person.

Most times, your doctor reassures you why every headache is not a red flag for a brain tumor, and why every chest pain is not signaling a heart attack. Most of the head pain you feel will occur with a perfectly normal brain. A brain scan will not add value when evaluating most headaches. Saving you and the state a dollar.

Importantly, all of your worries, concerns, fears, and expectations will come out spontaneously if your doctor is a big ear.

Unfortunately, sometimes the doctor takes your medical jargons as true and treats you based on the "diagnosis" that you provide. Tell the doc with certainty that you have stomach ulcers, and you may get treated for ulcers. Rather tell a simple story, "Doc, in the past, I was treated for ulcers and recovered. Now I have pain at the same spot, and it feels like that ulcer pain; I suspect that old problem." Your suspicion then does not throw doc off the right diagnostic pathway. Before giving you ulcer meds, your doc will first look for other medical monsters. Your stomach ulcers share symptoms with other monsters like stomach cancer, liver disease, pancreatic cancer, pancreatitis, or heart failure.

Sometimes the diagnosis you suspect is what the doctor also suspects; sometimes only one of you will be right! As you tell doc your fears and suspected diagnosis, the doctor has in the back of his or her mind the question "What else could this be?" The doc always thinks about all the possible diagnoses, including your suspected diagnosis.

## Question Time

By the time doc starts firing questions, you should have told him or her everything about your main symptom(s) in detail, your way. The doc usually confirms with you if symptom number one is, indeed, your main problem before firing more questions. Question time helps your doc to plug the gaps in your story about the primary symptom. Even if you listed multiple symptoms, your doctor picks only one that he or she thinks brought you consulting and asks detailed questions about it. If you give a minor problem first, your dollar is spent solving that problem.

The doc then asks more questions to clarify the main problem, like shortness of the breath:

"Besides passing urine frequently, have you also started drinking too much water?"

"Besides the swelling of your feet, has your tummy also started swelling or hurting lately?" "Have you noticed puffiness of your face in the mornings?"

"Do you get wheezing sounds in your chest from time to time?"

"Have you got an associated fever?"

All this time is spent on probing "shortness of the breath" and not on that rash, yet. Breathlessness was mentioned first and doc took it serious.

You will know it when you and your doc are on the same page; during question time, it starts to feel like "This doc seems to be reading my mind." Usually when you are done stating your case, the doctor would know what set of questions to ask. This depends on your main symptom and its other closely related symptoms and whether doc has been a good ear. Whenever doc starts "reading your mind," it means you have told your medical story well and your doc is a good listener.

As the *expert* who brings the health dollar, you should gently protest by nudging the doctor back to the main symptom, should he or she want to rush to other symptoms: "Doc, this pain in my chest is really what brought me in today; my knee can wait for another day." At any time during the consultation, you may interrupt the doc for clarity if he or she uses medical words that he or she wrongly assumes you know: "Doc, what do you mean by "inflammation"?"


Rearranging the ducks

"Oops, Doc, the swollen knee and painful eye are only part of the problems; pus discharge in my private parts is my major problem." These three seemingly diverse symptoms are indeed related, but the most worrying to this patient is the discharge. This patient does not lose too much because he quickly rearranged the symptoms in order of importance.

Your verbal hints and body language may alert the doctor that you arranged your problems the wrong way around. The doctor may then rearrange the consultation completely based on the newly identified main problem. You may not be so lucky to have a doctor get your ducks in a row for you. To overhaul the consultation, it may take an extra 50–75 percent of the time you have already spent. The doctor may charge you an extra health dollar for that, or the consultation may not be as thorough as for patients who put their ducks in a row right from the start.

If your ducks are lined in a row, you are unlikely to surprise your doc with: "Doc, what would be the best treatment for piles?" It is on your way out that you state what really brought you to consult: pain, swelling, or intense itching on the backside. You had withheld your main problem, painted a "migraine picture," and doc spent twenty minutes managing a minor headache. At that point, you might be told to make another appointment for the problem that really made you bring a dollar to doc. Another option would be to push you right back to the end of the queue for that day—your time, your dollar.

# Six

## Your Other Medical Symptoms
## (The Minor Ducks, the *Other Suspects*)

Your body has other organ systems that perform different functions and provide a hideout for minor symptoms, the other suspects. They all are portrayed by the third duck in the row. These symptoms may not have bothered you a lot, but you may feel that you should mention them, too. These are the symptoms that spoil the consultation for many patients. Patients compromise symptom number one by rushing the doctor through the long symptom list without spending enough time on the main problem.

The third duck in the row depicts your other favorite medical symptoms that existed before problem number one manifested. These other minor symptoms that would have messed up the earlier part of your consultation are discussed here. By now the main symptom should have been discussed well and thoroughly. Looked at as a duck in the row, this group of symptoms will only follow duck one and two, the main symptom and the story about that main symptom.

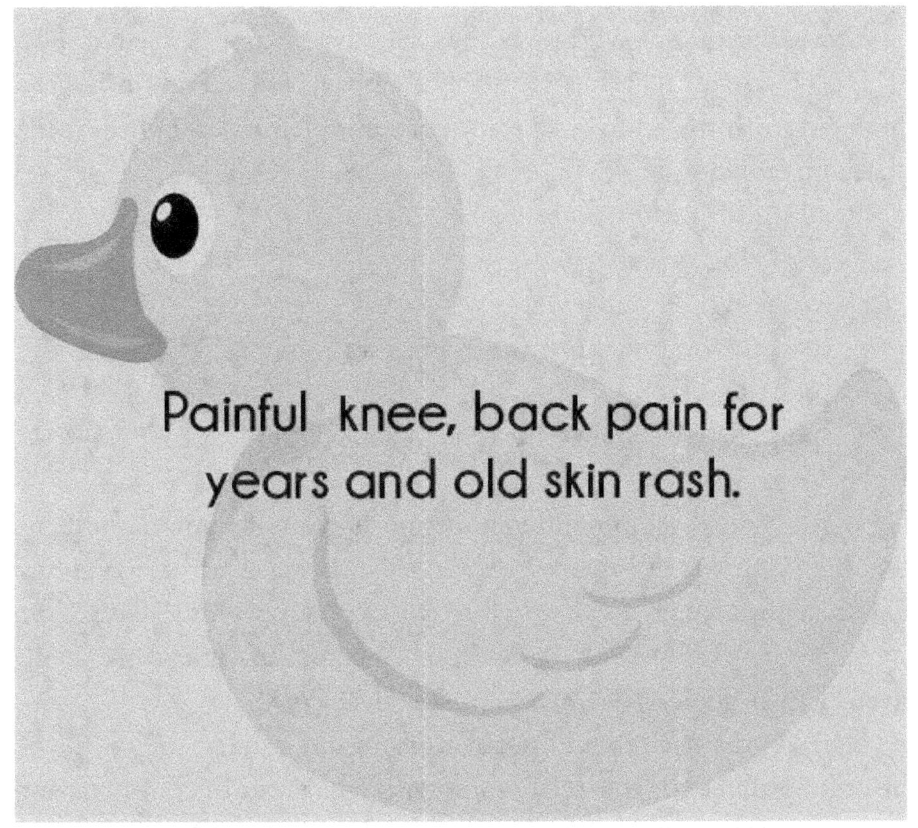


***Duck 3: symptoms that can mess up the story of breathlessness.
They have been around for some time. They can wait.***

If you started off well, then by this stage, both you and your doctor will know that this consultation dollar is well spent. On the other hand, if you misrepresented the main problem at the beginning, then both of you may want the consultation to end soon. You would think that this is a *bad doc*, and doc would think you are a *difficult patient*. With your health dollar wasted, you and the doctor will have had a lousy consultation, and you take home more pills and frustration than health. Doc also gets a headache when you leave.

This is a group of symptoms that may or may not be related to the main problem but that do arise from other parts of the body, other than the organ with the main symptom. For example, your weight loss may be accompanied by

- a roaring appetite;
- drinking too much water;
- passing too much urine, which leads to more thirst;
- blurring of your vision; or
- pins and needles in your feet.

These symptoms are from different organs in the body but may tell your doc that your weight loss may be due to your sugar factory gone bust. This diagnosis emerges long before the doc starts physically examining you. The diagnosis has come from your mouth, your story. Dollar saved. This is good *science and business of medicine*.

Do not push the other minor symptoms too fast, lest they will mask the main problem. If the doc does not ask you about those other symptoms, you can always bring them up after main problem is discussed well: "Doc, I do not know whether these are related to the main problem, but I have these other symptoms."

All the symptoms that you mention in this section are never probed in great detail like the main problem. Never drag a symptom from "your other medical problems list" to the "biggest symptom" part of your story. You have always had these symptoms but they never pushed you to see a doctor.

Sometimes what worries you as a disease entity is most likely another minor symptom that accompanies the main problem and is part of the final diagnosis. When the main problem is sorted, the minor symptoms fade away.

# Seven

## The Usual Suspects
## (Your Longstanding Health Problems)

Call these your permanent ducks in the pond (the usual suspects), because other symptoms/illnesses come and go, but these are medical problems that you have had (or will have) for a long time. When new symptoms have arisen in your body, it is not necessarily the usual suspects at fault. A duck that never leaves the pond is that kind of usual suspect; other ducks come and go but the usual suspects always remain in/around the pond. If the pond has been messed up then the regular duck takes the blame first. The same is true for a disease that you have had for years. Hypertension can cause a headache, but it is not always the reason for every headache in a hypertensive patient. Asthma usually causes chest symptoms, but it is not the cause of every chest pain and breathlessness in an asthmatic person.

This part of your medical story looks at all of the

- past and longstanding illnesses;
- previous operations, medical procedures, blood transfusions, and transplants;

- allergies to medications, foods, or stings;
- past hospitalizations and reasons for these; and
- other remedies that you are using, however trivial.

(A special part of this is dedicated to women only).

All health problems that you might have had, or still have, shall be covered here by your doctor. The initial consultation may only skim through these problems, but in later consultations, the doctor will keep on asking you about these. If your past illnesses are the reason for your consultation today, then mention that first.

These usual suspects are depicted here by the fourth duck.

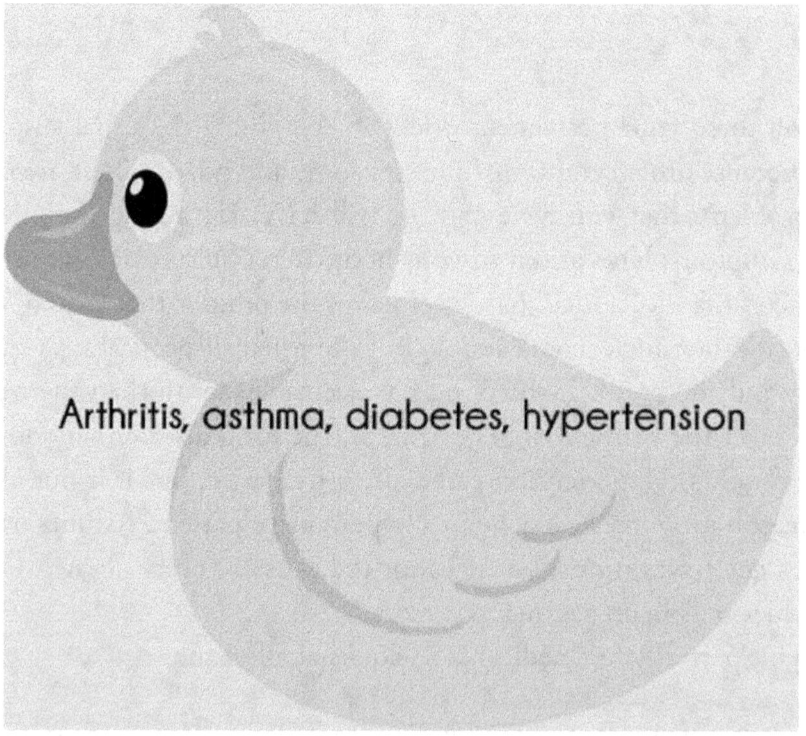



*Duck 4 depicts the usual suspects—always there with any new symptoms. Always there when the new symptoms are gone. This is the duck that hangs around the pond always.*

## Past Medical History

Some patients use these chronic illnesses to test the skills of a new doctor. They hide the known diagnoses from the new doctor intentionally. With time (and some dollars later), the new doctor will eventually discover the problems. This may be during the first consultation, or three consultations later. Only then do the patients reveal, "I forgot to tell you, Doc—I have been taking these thyroid medications for the past ten years." Diagnostic skills of the doctor were tested, but time and dollars wasted.

This is an expensive way to test the skills of your new doctor. You wouldn't want to pay for the extra (unnecessary) tests and time taken for the doctor to discover the old diagnosis that you already know about. Time wasted on reinventing the wheel (rediscovering your old diagnosis) is time you pay for. Save yourself time, pain (unnecessary needle pricks), and a dollar.

Revealing all your past medical problems helps you get better health at every consultation. Some patients prefer to start their storytelling by giving their past medical history, and it is advantageous. It grabs the doctor's attention at the beginning, and he or she will know that you are serious about the business that brought you in that day. It also sets a good background for stating the number-one problem.

This is also your chance to tell the doctor which medications have worked in the past and which ones have not worked to treat your chronic illnesses.

Descriptions of previous hospital admissions and reasons for the hospitalizations give your doc inside info and help him or her to treat you like an insider. Once your doctor knows about all the past and present medications that you have used or are using, it allows him or her to prescribe carefully. You help yourself by helping the doc with info.

Once you have given your doctor your past medical problems, then you may proceed straight to the problem of the day.

The story line may go, "Doc, I have had type two diabetes for ten years. I take *metformin* and *gliclazide*. I am allergic to penicillin. Generally I have been in good health over the past nine years. *Now, what brings me to consult today is* this throbbing headache affecting the left side of my face, and my left nostril is blocked." Although the headache is mentioned after the past medical history, it will be clear to the doctor that it is the main problem. Not all patients can tell their story this way, but it does not matter. You can always start your story with problem number one as described earlier. *Acute rhino-sinusitis* is the *visiting* diagnosis, but diabetes is the old problem and not at fault this time. When the acute problem is cured, the diabetes stays and goes nowhere. It is a permanent resident.

Different medications in your drug cabinet sit separately from one another in little bottles, but once they are inside your body, all medications sit in one *big bottle*. Once absorbed into your body, the medications find their way into your bloodstream and form one large soup of pills that interact with each other, with food, and even with sunlight. Some medications dilute the effects of other medications, while some medications work together to kill you.

Common examples are as follows:

- Different medications meant for different diseases could work together to lower your blood pressure dangerously, causing death.
- Medicines from two different drug classes could together cause severe elevation of your blood pressure, and even a stroke.
- If a man who has taken potency pills has a heart attack, he may require medication that improves blood flow to the heart but that might cause a fatal drop in his blood pressure. These are two drugs that work in two different systems, but together they can kill you. The two drugs work in organs that are miles apart, but they get to "talk to each other" inside your body and may "plot" to harm you. Tell your doc about all your meds.

- A failing heart can also produce asthma-like symptoms, and some pills used to treat heart failure also worsen asthma symptoms. Even if the Internet tells you that you have asthma, let your doc know that you also have hypertension or heart disease in the background.

These are the advantages of telling your doctor about every pill that you take, even if it is just a vitamin. The symptoms about which you have come to consult may be the side effects of some of the pills that you take. Some of your symptoms are caused by your diseases, and some of the symptoms may be caused by the pills that "fix" those diseases. Instead of the doc giving you pills to move your bowels, he or she might help you by stopping/changing one or two of your current meds. Drugs can interact by fighting one another instead of fighting the disease.

Do not only name the big-ticket pills, like those for heart disease and diabetes. This list should include medicines bought over the counter without a prescription and medications from friends or family. Do not forget to mention your herbal teas and other natural products in this list. Natural products are also medications, although acquired without a prescription. As an example, when taking St. John's wort together with the antidepressant, Prozac, you could potentially overdose on the same ingredient from two different products.

## Past Surgical History

This could affect the treatment of the current disease, or the disease could have an effect on you based on the past surgery. This includes the following:

- Past surgical treatments or operations, both major and minor. If you have been under the knife, please tell the doc.

- Major injuries in the past. It might have seemed minor to you, but report it if you remember.
- Any organ transplantation that you may have received or any organ that you may have donated to someone else.
- Blood transfusion or infusion of other blood products. Some diseases are a result of transfusion of blood or blood products.
- Being examined with tubes with small cameras (endoscopes) pushed into a body orifice and any biopsies taken.

### *Past Gynecological History and Past Obstetric History*

This part of medical history (*her* story) applies to women only. Doctors are crazy about the first day of the last month during which a lady gets her periods. Such intimate details will help your doctor

- to exclude or confirm the possibility of a pregnancy as this changes the way your doc prescribes;
- to know how your biological clock is ticking;
- to know if a gynecological disorder has set in;
- to deduce if a woman's prolonged and heavy menstrual flow is related to the blood-thinning drug she is on; or
- to know if some tumors have invaded the body.

Patients with a bleeding disorder may flow too heavily and too frequently. Very heavy menstrual flow may be related to the dizzy spells, shortness of breath, leg swelling, fatigue, and chest pain for which a woman consults.

Women have a different and very unique biological makeup and subsequently different biological challenges. Although the word "men" is integral to some of the gynecological terms, these words have nothing to do with the male gender: *men*orrhagia (abnormal heavy menstrual flow), a*men*orrhea (absence or lack of menstruation), dys*men*orrhea (painful *men*struation), poly*men*orrhea (irregular, multiple, and abnormal menstrual flows per month), *men*arche (first *men*struation), and *men*opause (when menstrual flows come to a permanent stop). This terminology is preserved for women only, because men already have a prostate to nurse! These are part of the possible usual suspects for the female patient.

The fetus of a pregnant woman gets to share all the medicines that she takes, so does a baby on the breast. If a there is a baby in the tummy or breastfeeding, let your doc know before you even sit down. Whatever a breastfeeding mother eats or drinks, the baby sucks in the breast milk. Again remind the doc when getting your prescription.

These gynecological events and the times they occur give your doc clues about your breast, bone, blood, ovarian, and womb health. These events and their timing may also be influenced by your current pill use, jabs, or implants/gynecological devices. Missed periods may influence a doctor's prescribing habits for a woman of reproductive age. A hysterectomy also changes the way your doc prescribes.

# Eight

## HABITS, HOBBIES, AND OCCUPATION

By the time your story starts moving toward your habits/hobbies, you and your doc shall have thoroughly discussed the main symptom, other symptoms, and the usual/old medical problems.

A doctor who asks about these private issues is not prying. The little things that we do can affect how medications work in the body. These things that we do for pleasure or pain bring forth good health or ill health.

### Habits and hobbies

Pleasurable habits may cause pain in the long run. Some painful habits, like exercise, are taxing at the beginning but relieve pain and suffering in the long run. Knowledge of your habits helps your doctor in making a diagnosis and planning your treatment. Included here are the following:

- Cigarettes, alcoholic drinks, coffee, and soft drugs (Coffee can also cause symptoms or interact with some medications)
- Exercise or the lack of it
- Outings or the lack thereof

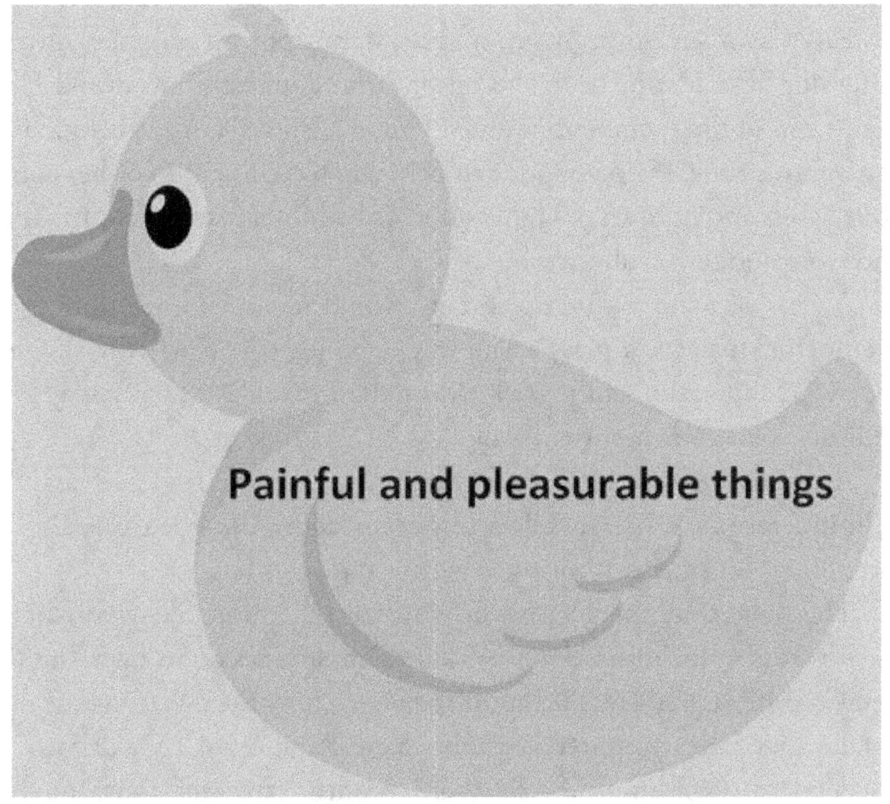


***Duck 5: things that we do for pleasure or for pain.***

Regarding exercise:

Do you irritate the neighborhood dogs by walking around the block five times a week? Do you frequently venture into the bush or climb hills?

These are all examples of close encounters with nature and are good for your overall health. Any physical activity that raises our heart rates takes us back to our cave days, but instead of being an escape from predators, exercise helps us escape from some medical monsters. The escape always feels good, and that is what exercise does.

Fever, swollen groin gland, and an itchy spot on your leg on the same side after a stint in to the bush? A random tick bite would have tried to spoil the therapeutic value of your bush walk. Your habits help at diagnosis time. Help your doc to help you by telling him or her about your habits and hobbies, whether good or bad. Doc also has some habits and won't judge you about yours.

A glass of wine with a meal daily would not send you running to the doctor. Instead, a glass a day might be just the medicine the doc ordered. Moderation is the trick. More than two glasses daily may give your doc some business eventually.

A sedentary lifestyle may feel good now, but the trade-off may be pain in later years. Meanwhile a physically active lifestyle earlier in life looks like a lot of effort but the payoff is big years later.

The more time the TV spends with you, the more likely you are to visit doctors in the future. The TV causes no illnesses on its own, but the many uninterrupted and idle hours spent watching the TV, using the digital device, or the computer are problematic. An hour of TV a day would not send you consulting the following month. However, four hours of television daily may harm you over years. Moderation is the solution.

A regular walk around the block or out of your comfort zone

- makes your doctor's prescription shorter and less frequent;
- makes for a shorter and cheaper consultation (your doctor does not have to preach to you about its benefits);
- improves your health in all the vital domains; and
- makes your visits to the doctor less frequent, and you are more likely to meet your doc jogging than in his or her rooms.

Physical exercise in any form is a type of calculated risk, and besides you push your body through the tasks it was meant to do. The benefits of calculated risks usually seem to outweigh the losses thereof. The automobile has taken over the functions of the multiple joints that we were created with. Regular walks will make you regain some of your bodily functions. Exercise pushes you to break barriers that the world sets for you. The more brisk walks you take, the more you may discover that you are the "world" and that you have set those barriers yourself.

If you still have any parts of your body that you can move, let that be your exercise and do it regularly.

Going out into the *wild*, even if it is just in the town park, exposes us to the simplicity and sophistication of life away from the complexity of concrete jungle. That brief exposure to nature allows your body and mind to be in one place at the same moment—the art of being present. Sedentary life style messes up the way your body functions, health fades, and your dollar follows the fading health. Besides, being out of the house alone gets your heart and joints moving faster with big benefits to your well-being. Getting out of the house on foot also exposes you to some form of *wilderness*; the people you drive past daily seem so different and tame when you walk past them. You miss a whole universe when you do not get to experience your hood on foot.

Other pills work well only once the disease has found a home in your body or mind; exercise is a pill that may work well before, or after the disease gets established. Hard-work-without-pay is a pill that you get for free and helps keep you and your dollar away from doc; it prevents many an ailment. Few ailments mean few visits to doctors. Coin saved.


*Occupation*

"But really, Doc, what does my job have to do with my heartburn?"

Almost no job is without occupational hazards; ask your doc about the hazards of jobs in the field of medicine. The hazards that come with being a doctor are numerous. When a doctor treats another doc, he or she sees a patient at high risk for burnout, addiction, stress, anxiety, depression, compassion fatigue, and a higher-than-normal rate of suicide. Your job must also have its own hazards, may be fewer than ours.

When a herdsman comes in with a fever to see his doctor and never mentions his occupation, he delays the process of arriving at a diagnosis. A coal miner who goes to consult for a cough and hides his or her occupation surely does not want a quick diagnosis. Almost every occupation out there has its benefits and hazards.

A job that you do just for the money is bound to make you ill. Lucky are those who get paid for having fun: musicians, athletes, and artists. Always aim at getting paid for having fun. Let your doc know how much you love or hate your job. A job that you need but resent is bound to hurt you, but one that you love and are passionate about is bound to keep you healthy, besides giving you a paycheck. Your job, thus, can hurt or heal you.

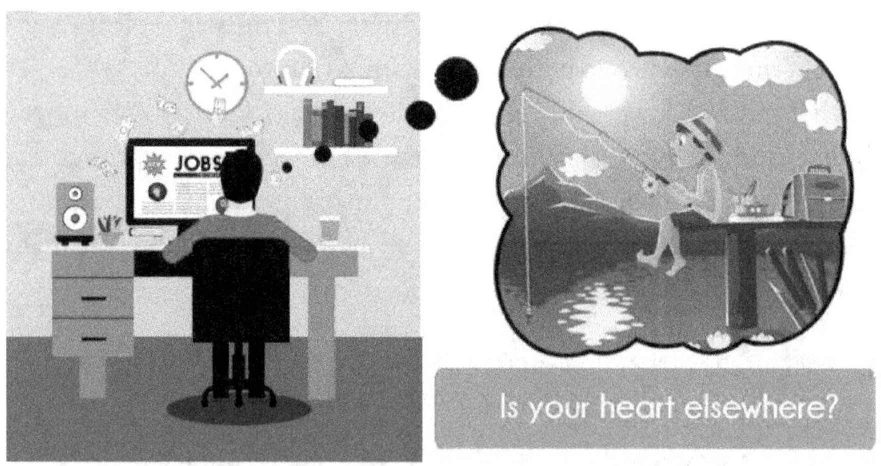

# Nine



## Your Crowd
### (Story about the People Who Make You)

The Creator *created* you; the people whom you live with and encounter daily are the ones who *make* you. Who you are now is because of who your crowd was yesterday, and who you will be tomorrow is determined by your current crowd.

Believe it or not, some aspects of your family composition and structure determine your state of well-being or ill health. Your family is very efficient at giving you good health, and it is equally effective at causing you ill health. Your family is both a bug and a pill in that respect, depending on the factors at play at specific times.

Each family member normally gives all the other family members either heaven or hell, depending on the clock. Every family member has a duty of giving or receiving heaven or hell; that is what a perfect family does. In spite of all this, your family is just perfect like the other families out there.

So when asked about family, do not paint a rosy picture; give your doctor the real picture including all the roses and all the thorns. Your

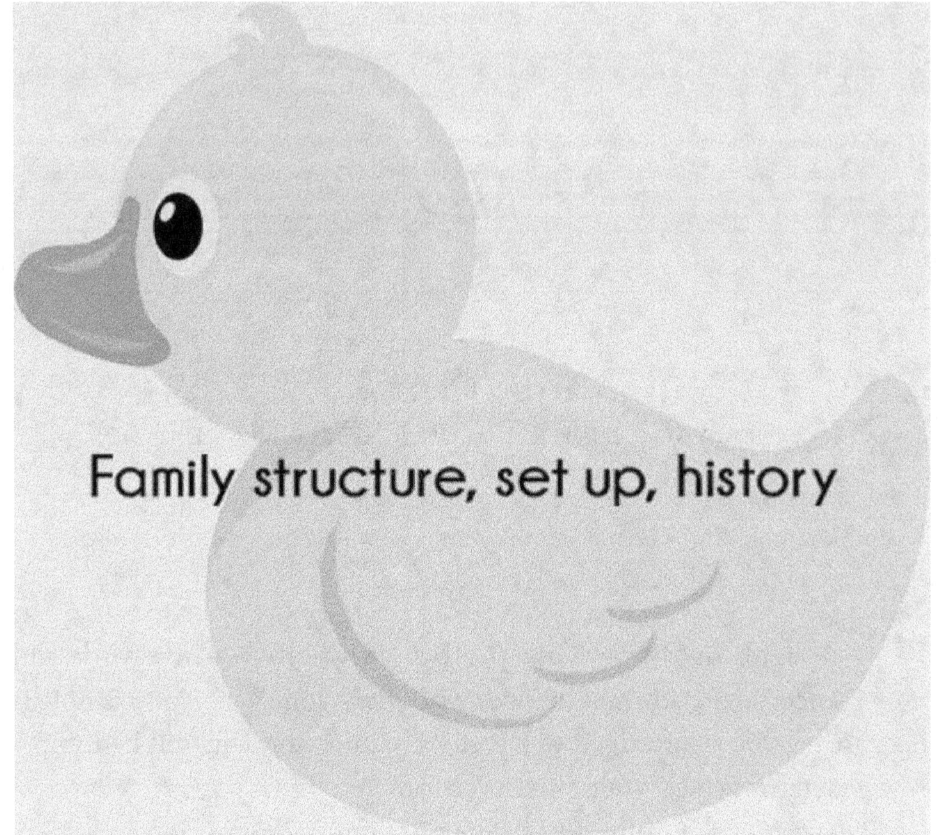


**Duck 6: talks about your immediate crowd and the bigger crowd out there.**

doctor has heard worse family stories than yours. If you fear scaring your doctor on the first day of the consultation, do tell them more during later consultations. Any part of your family life that interferes with your sleep can interfere with your health. Whoever or whatever makes you lose sleep will invariably cause you some sort of pain.

Indeed, human beings are *hurting* beings. The hurt that you get from a tongue-lashing may be worse than being mauled by a lion. The wounds of a sharp tongue run deep and take years to heal. Walking among us are *hurt beings*. Worse still, they do not receive the sympathy that the one mauled by a lion gets, for they have no visible wounds or scars. As much as we hurt others, we are also *healing* beings. The touch of our hands, words of sympathy, our empathy, our tears, and just being there for a friend are all powerful drugs.

Do not be surprised if you consult for a cough that has lasted for weeks and your doctor is more interested in finding out whether

- any of your family member suffers from hay fever;
- any of your kids or adult relatives have longstanding rash, darkening and itching of the skin; and
- some in your family have stubborn red and itchy eyes.

The symptoms that your family members have may help your doctor to quickly discover that you have asthma. During this part of the interview, *innocent* members of your family are *dragged* into the consultation.

Even if the doctor hasn't asked, talk about your family if it bothers you. Your doctor is not only interested in body-based problems. Dysfunctional families cause ill health just as malfunctioning organs or tissues. Because your story does not sound *medical* is not a problem as far as doc, the listener, is concerned. Your doc makes medical diagnoses out of *nonmedical stories*. You may just be the *symptom of a family problem*; the family may be the unit in need of healing, and you are the big story (the first symptom) of the family problem.

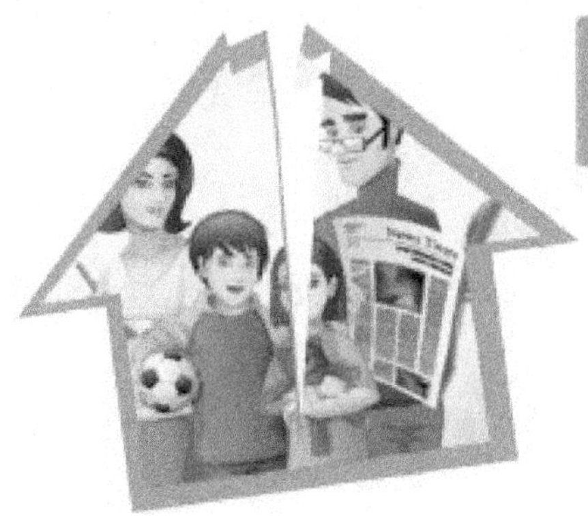

Family getting torn apart? This story is as important as the chest pain that took you to consult, may be more. Let your doc know about such things.

Health gets torn apart when family is torn apart. The doc may not fix the disruption all the time, but he or she can fix the illnesses that accompany these issues.

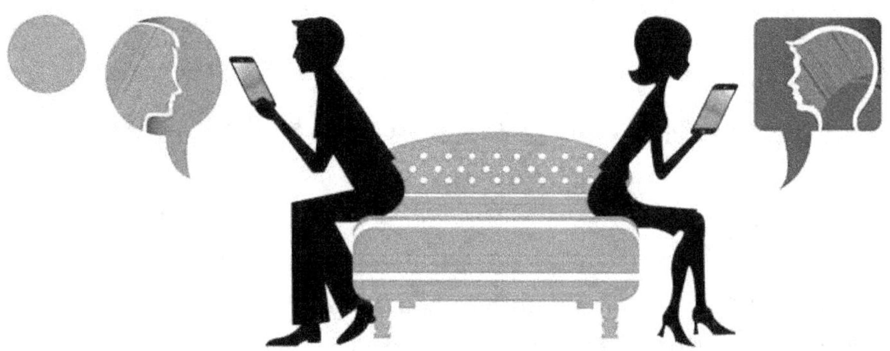

Do you spend more time sharing with your digital family in the virtual world than with the real family with whom you share physical space? The health of the family members who live with you may take a knock or a boost, depending on the dynamics of the things you do online and the time you spend with your online family. The time your family spends online may also affect your health. It is good for your doctor to know the balance you strike between *time spent online* and *time spent on earth*.

## Uprooting

Take anyone from a familiar environment, and put him or her in a new environment, and the person's state of health changes, short or long term. The change in his or her health status may be negative or positive.

Few people are not affected by uprooting. Marriage, separation, divorce, transfers, new jobs, job loss, and evictions are forms of uprooting.

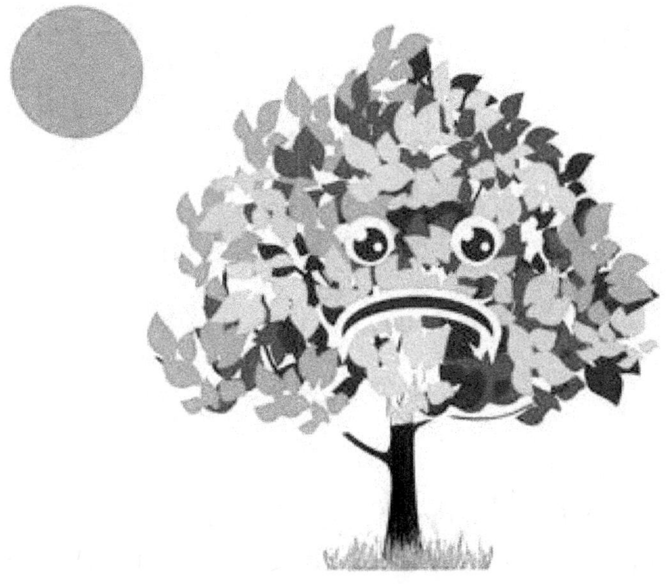

Uproot a tree from a rain forest, plant
it in the desert, and see if it enjoys
great health. Likewise, a desert palm tree
may not thrive with the abundant water supply in the
rain forests.

# Ten

## Physical Examination
## (The Search for Evidence)

Invasive as it may feel, physical examination should never be a violation of your privacy and personhood. You can always choose to have a chaperone present during an examination. This keeps inappropriate doctors in check and limits false accusations, but it comes with loss of confidentiality. Physical examinations are invasive; even a simple act of *opening your mouth wide* is invasive. If you are not comfortable with the consultation, do not get onto that exam table! Indeed, if you are uncomfortable with your doctor, terminate the consultation during the story time. Ethics requires all doctors to treat you and the consultation with utmost respect and professionalism.

If during the physical medical examination it starts to feel like "This doc really knows what he or she is looking for," it means that

- you have told a good story and you have been a good artist;
- your medical ducks were lined up in a row;
- your doc has been a big ear;

- your doc is book worm; he or she has had a good training and keeps abreast with his or her science; or
- the business of medicine will be stacked in your favor.

Physical examination is not just a random science of medical hammers, lights, percussion, and the stethoscope but there is also an art in that. Even outside the medical consultation, artists and scientists add some beauty to the world. You and doctor both bring some beauty into a medical consultation, you bring the art and doc brings the science.

Some forms of examination may feel downright childish, but this is no game time. Looking for a plantar reflex in the soles of your feet is an example of nervous-system examination that tickles most people. A search for swollen glands in your armpits may make you wonder what is wrong with your doc. An examination does not give permission to doctors to behave inappropriately. Examination entails assessing you holistically. You and doc can also discuss bowling or golf during physical examination.

There is a lot about you that doc and his or her tools can never unearth. It is your duty to volunteer such info. Sometimes it feels rather silly bringing your work-related issues during physical examination, but some of those *silly issues* could make or break the consultation. You may be surprised at how important your doctor will find such info to be. Nonmedical info that you bring up very late in the consultation is sometimes what makes you get the best out of your health dollar. Story time never ends when you are being examined.

The patient depicted below has a long list of nonmedical problems, which he shares with his doc and gets a very good medical consultation at the end.

Such private, *unimportant* areas of your life may hide medically important info. Such nonmedical talk helps direct doc to which organs

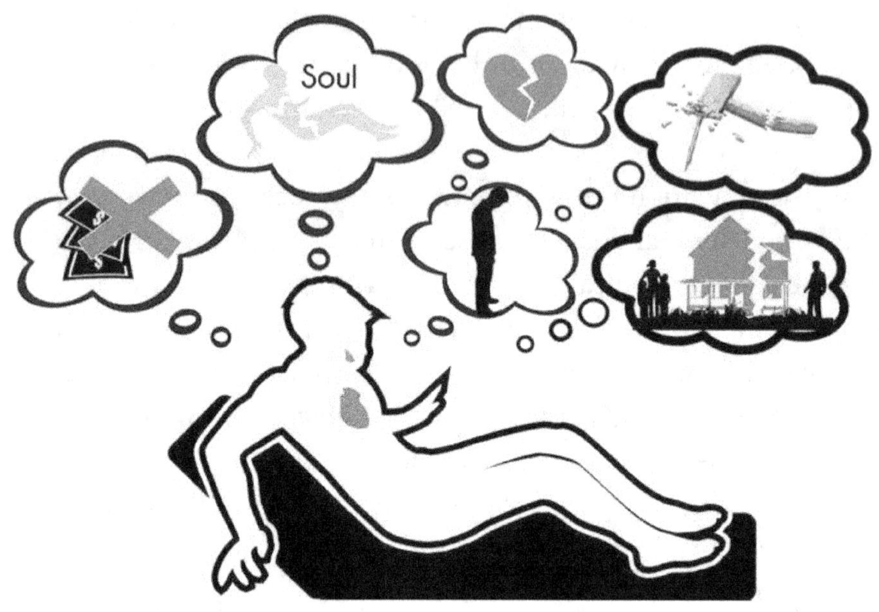


to examine well, preventing some expensive medical tests and scans—a buck saved.

If your chest pain got worse the day you witnessed your workmate complain of chest pain and die within minutes, or if it got worse the month your younger brother survived a heart attack, tell your doc. This story may come while you are getting off the examination table, but it helps your doctor save you a health dollar.

Physical examination includes inspecting your body, palpating (touching or handling), percussing (gently making a "drum" of your tummy or chest), and auscultation (listening with the stethoscope.)

- Indecent touch is not part of a physical examination; it is a criminal offence.
- Indecent remarks by a doc during a physical examination are unethical and criminal.

- Overexposure of areas not being examined is not acceptable; the exception is for parts that are already exposed when you walk into the consultation. Only limited parts of your body should be exposed as the examination progresses. Areas already examined are covered while the doc proceeds to examine other parts of your body. Sometimes a large part of the body may need to be briefly exposed for doc to get a bird's eye view of a disease.

Fortunately, word of mouth puts the unprofessional doctor out of business or in jail. Asking around before you choose a doc is a dollar and life saver.

## *The Mind May Be Outside the "Brain Box"*

Your brain is a thing confined in a box (the skull). The cables and chemicals that may explain the functioning of the mind are inside that brainbox, but the mind may be a thing found outside that brainbox. If the mind is in the confines of the brainbox then it is hard to see. Doctors cannot see your mind on brain scans. The physical examination, scans, and other tests do not help your doc find what is on your mind; you help your doc do that.

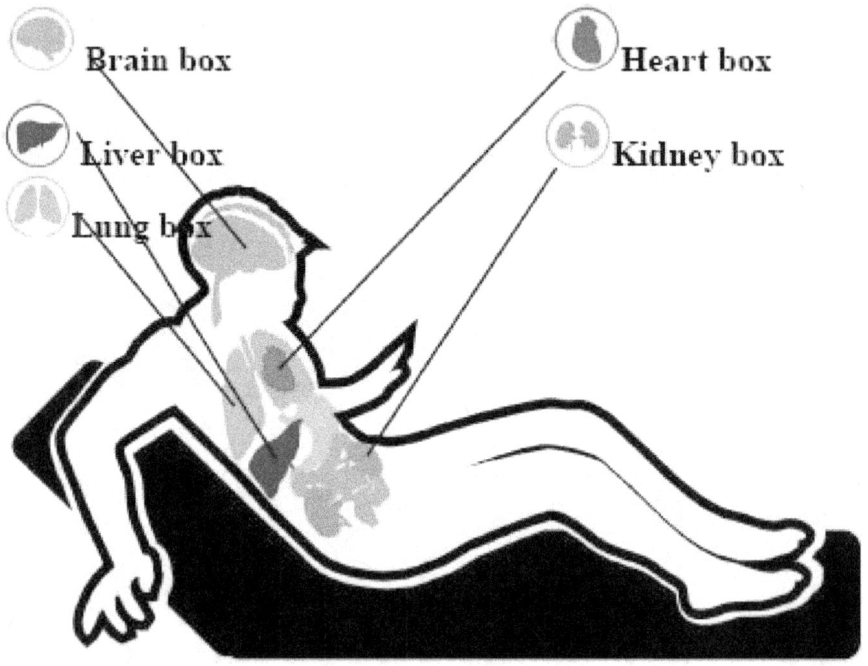


*This patient has not come to see the doctor; he has just brought his organs to the doctor. He expects orgnan-specific diagnosis to be found and cured. He hasn't let the doc into his life, family, work, "heart," and mind. He gave a disease-specific story. He wants disease-specific answers. Don't be this kind of patient. He seems to have no room for an illness, just diseases only.*

Some patients take a chest pain to the doctor and expect a disease to be found inside the chest and removed; they seek a cure. Wrong, because sometimes the pain in the chest is caused by an illness. Unlike diseases, illnesses leave no medical footprints that can be seen on scans. Tuberculosis of the lungs, for example, is a disease that leaves significant medical evidence (footprints) that are found on examination of the body, sputum, tissues, and x-rays. This is why a physical examination might find *nothing wrong* in someone who has multiple symptoms. Just like a person with tuberculosis, one with an illness is equally unwell, or even worse off, but with no medical evidence on examination and tests.

## Inspection

The doc may surprise you at this point. He or she may peer at a part of your body with such great intent that you feel he or she has forgotten about the rest of you. This is an important part of information gathering that sometimes doctors skip or skillfully integrate in the consultation such that you may not notice. The inspection starts as you walk in and while the doctor is listening to your story.

This may be a simple look at your tummy with the doc's eyes at the same level or the doc standing next to you. It has big implications if you have been vomiting some green stuff and have severe abdominal pain. The same is done during an examination of your chest. Your doctor is not wasting your time with such seemingly bizarre moves. It might save you some health dollars, because such simple maneuvers could exclude the use of costly tests. Some treatment may even start before the x-rays are done. It does you no good for the doctor to rush to the stethoscope.

## Palpation

In lay terms, this is when the doctor touches or handles parts of your body in a professional manner to look for physical signs of disease. Inappropriate touching is not palpation. There should be gentleness and caution during palpation. Prodding and poking are not part of palpation. Your doctor normally asks you to point out the most painful areas so that they are palpated last and with caution. Palpation helps doc to identify tender areas. Medically, *tenderness* refers to pain induced by touch or handling. Forget about the *tenderness* of your steak or partner.

## Percussion

This is reminiscent of a musical instrument called the percussion, and when we percuss your tummy or chest, we are saving your life and also making musical moments out of your medical misery! This is not for fun, but it can help us arrive at a diagnosis before blood tests and costly scans. The doc places one hand flat on your body and hammers the middle finger of the flat hand with the middle finger of the other hand; the sound produced is a diagnostic gold mine.

This is not game time. It can help your doctor quickly come to a conclusion as to whether your severe abdominal pain is related to a perforated intestine or an obstructed one. Both are surgical emergencies that require rapid response to minimize complications, or even death.

So the next time your doctor turns your tummy or chest into a drum (percussion) for a minute, let him or her be your guest! Your doc may not win a musical Grammy award, though.

This is a simple part of the examination that can save a dollar on tests.

## Auscultation

The history of medicine has a story on how a doc improvised a stethoscope. Doctors of days gone by would listen to the heart and lungs by awkwardly placing an ear on the patient's chest. This quickly changed when a doc had to examine the wife of an important man in the presence of a chaperone, the husband himself. The quick-thinking doc reportedly rolled a piece of paper into a tube, put its one end on the lady's chest, and listened through the other end of the tube; a tool was born. The sound quality was even better, the doc's head was at a safe distance from the lady's chest, and from problems. (I am not certain whether this event involved Dr Laenec, or some other doctor and then Dr Laenec made the tool famous).

This may be the most colorful part of the examination for many patients, but by the time the stethoscope comes off the doctor's neck and onto your chest, the diagnosis will have been clinched much earlier. Your story would have given your doc the diagnosis, some of the times. Some medical specialties do not even require the stethoscope at all; some require it all the time.

Most patients feel robbed if a consultation ends without the mighty tube landing on their chests. For many, this seems to be the tube that tells all to the doctor. But remember that not everything that is happening on the inside can be heard through the stethoscope. Most times, your story is more important. If there was a way of putting the stethoscope on a patient's mouth to get the full medical history straight from the source, we would avoid many tests.

## Major Exam Points

You shall have thrown your health dollar to the docs if you withhold some parts of your body, feelings, and thoughts from the examining doctor. Your diagnosis hides in bizarre places.

Big emphasis: do not climb onto the examination table of a doctor you are not comfortable with. Do not even walk into the consultation room if for any reason, you do not trust or like the doctor. Physical examination can be intimate, but intimate examinations are key to picking out some common forms of dangerous cancers in both sexes.

A detailed and accurate story is more important than the physical examination most of the time. If you played around during story time, you might as well have played with your health dollar. If your storytelling was accurate, the physical examination will be focused on organs that your story clarified to the doctor. Many doctors rush to do the physical examination after a very brief interview. For many patients, not much may be gained during this part of the assessment (except during medical emergencies). This point stresses the importance of making sure that the few words that come out of your mouth contain the most vital symptoms of the day.

Making a diagnosis is not possible most of the time; with many diseases/illnesses, the doctor finds nothing wrong during physical examination. Because nothing abnormal was found during examination does not mean that there is nothing wrong with you. Your doc can still come up with a package of your problems and labels them as an *assessment*, not just one medical diagnostic label with a Latin or Greek name. The *blah-blah syndrome* is a disease label that many patients would rather take home than *generalized anxiety disorder*.

If your diagnosis turns out to be "There is nothing wrong with you," it could be due to the fact that your doctor concentrated only on examining your flesh, the part of you that gets on the examination table. Many times, as doctors, we give little attention to *you* (the real you). This means that the doc does not give attention to

- your heart—this is different to the one that pumps blood, this is the one that *pumps tears* and emotions. It is the heart that cardio-thoracic surgeons cannot see when they open a chest during surgery;

- your mind—the thing that sits outside the brainbox (or could it be inside the brainbox);
- your ego;
- what makes you to be *you*—that part of you that "floats above the examination table," the part that you cannot describe well. In fact I (as a doctor) do not know what it is and where it sits in you;
- your crowd and your "castle"—your human environment;
- your work environment; or
- your pocket and financial environment—issues of the wallet or purse.

When you lie on that table, the doctor mostly examines only your body and brain plus the rest of the nervous system. Examining your central nervous system (brain, spine, and nerves) tells your doctor little or nothing about your mind (mental health). Your story gives doc a lot more about your mental, emotional, economic, social, and spiritual well-being than the examination.

Examination time is still story time. Some patients save the most important or "shameful" part of storytelling for this part of the consultation. This is the time some patients drop the bombshell: "Doc, my wife just packed and left with the kids last month," or "Doc, I think my husband has started seeing his ex-wife again."

You might bring this up toward the very end of the consultation, but this is actually what brought you to the consultation in the first place. It may come late but it is still your first duck. It will save you a lot on painful and costly investigations or costly and dangerous medications. This also saves you from unnecessary referrals to other health-care providers. This is a part of the assessment that does not require you to rehearse how you respond to the evaluation.

*Tips*

- Whenever your doctor touches (palpates) parts of your body, do not act out "ouch" if there is no pain. Do not try to be a good patient and give the doctor what you think he or she needs from you. Most times, if he or she does not tell you to do anything, it means just that: you do not have to do anything.

- When you say "ouch" when there is no pain, you are bound to get wrong tests done, and your health dollar pays for the unnecessary tests ordered. You also get exposed to unnecessary treatment for that "ouch," and you also pay for it anyway.

- When your doctor hits your knee with a medical hammer, for example, you are not expected to give a kick in response. If you voluntarily help the doc by kicking, you hide the real response that the doctor is looking for, hence hiding your illness or falsely generating a disease that you don't have, and you end up getting treatment that you don't need.

- If possible, don't let your family or friends crowd the doctor in; this can cause problems. One or two family members may accompany you into the consultation, but avoid bringing a busload. Privacy is lost, and your doctor, once crowded in, may develop performance anxiety. Performing under pressure is not good for your doc and your health. While doctors may keep confidential all the information that you have given, your crowd may not have such professional obligation.

- If you cannot resist the urge to check your smartphone for the most recent postings, do not do it during your story time. You might just waste a lot of dollars in return for little health.

- However brief the physical examination is, it can reveal a lot of medical info to help your doctor arrive at a diagnosis. Sometimes it can be as brief as the doctor leaving his or her seat and coming to your side for a minute. This can happen when you have arranged your ducks (symptoms) in an orderly way and the doctor has made the diagnosis from the time you were telling your story (history).

### What is wrong with these doctors?

Some of the things the doctor does to you or asks you to do during a physical exam may be hilarious and make for a good laugh. Imagine doc puts a palm on your chest and asks you to say "ninety-nine" many times while he or she alternately touches either side of your chest. Later on, the doc auscultates your chest and again tells you to repeat the play stuff: "ninety-nine, ninety-nine, ninety-nine." You may be surprised at the amount of information the doctor can obtain from this little game of "ninety-nine"—whether one of your lungs has too much scar tissue, too much or too little air, or more fluid collection than the other.

Don't even think of laughing at the games that doctors play. "Open wide"—the doc means your mouth! What is wrong with these doctors? Even if it is a broken bone in your leg, you will always be asked to open wide. Surprise, surprise: this gives clues to doctors as to how much blood you lost in that broken bone and how easy (or hard) the anesthetist's work will be. You may be breathless and with swollen legs, and doc would still want you to open wide; a blue discoloration of your tongue, lips, and the inner lining of your mouth may confirm the diagnosis of heart failure. The open mouth may also tell doc about state of your liver and immune system. Now open wide again—in awe.

# Eleven

## The Politics of Medicine

During the interview, questions that can cause unease are related to the following:

- Ethnicity: it is a pity that some medical problems are "racist" in their patterns; there is a genetic and racial predisposition to some medical problems. Your ethnicity can help point where the doc should hunt for a diagnosis.
- Belief system: blood transfusions are a no-go area for one belief system. Some religions have a gender preference for the examining doctor. Wanting to know your religious affiliation is not an indication of prejudice. It is good for your health and improves the relationship between you and your doc.
- Physical address: just knowing where you reside can help your doc to narrow the diagnostic possibilities. Some medical problems even prefer specific street addresses, without the help of a GPS. Every little detail about your environment helps with the diagnosis.

- Your family structure, setup, and history could explain some symptoms better than a chest x-ray, EKG, heart sonar, or tests on your blood. Coin saved.
- Ethics.

Saying "ah" or "eh" gives the doc a good view of your throat, aiding in the diagnosis. Try this by opening your mouth in front of the mirror, first without making any sound and then while saying "ah" or "eh." You will be surprised at how much of your throat you can see. So now you know that saying "ah" is indeed not a joke. I bring this up because adult patients do not like it any one bit; they just stick the tongue out and open mouth without any "ah" or "eh." The open mouth is a diagnostic gold mine: whether talking or just wide open.

When we want to make fun of anyone, we make fun of other doctors, and Medicine has a gold mine of jokes about doctors for doctors. When the doc asks you to say "eh," he or she means serious medical business, trying to save your health dollar by making a diagnosis based mainly on your story and examination without many tests. This helps you avoid pain in your pocket and flesh. What sounds like game time is medical science. This is part of the politics of buying and selling health indeed; play the politics well and your dollar buys you a lot of health!

A brief, seemingly disrespectful pull on your eyelid may offend you. This simple "offense" could be a lifesaver. By that your doctor can quickly tell whether you have

- a badly behaving liver;
- a pancreas that interferes with the daily job of the liver;
- leaking blood taps (anemia of blood loss); or
- a blood factory that is asleep (anemia due to bone marrow at fault).

Your doc may press your ankle like someone uninterested in helping you, yet he or she is checking for the cause of the breathlessness that you reported. This may confirm whether your frequent urination at night could indeed be related to a failing heart.

Sometimes you may get angry that despite your struggle to breathe, the doctor only checked your pulse, looked hard at your fingernails, touched your chest, looked at your neck, pressed your ankle, and declared that you had heart failure. The examination may nauseate you, but it gives the doc so much health info.

To paint, or not to paint. If you love having painted nails, it might be a good idea to leave one nail unpainted when going to see a doc. This unpainted nail is a window to your inside. The nail can tell your doc about

- your gut health;
- your liver and pancreas health, or lack thereof;
- the health of your heart and lungs;
- your joint and bone health; and
- your nutritional state plus much more.

"And you won't believe it! This doctor just pressed my ankle, told me to stick out my tongue, poked at my tummy, took a casual look at my nails, and told me a lot of stuff about my liver. To say the least, I walked out of that room very dissatisfied." Such stories are common, but that basic, lackluster examination is a diagnostic treasure chest for your doc.

A painted lip during a medical examination? I have no idea whether it is a hindrance or not. But remember: the diagnosis comes from your mouth (story time and an opened mouth) plus inspection of the lips. The open but silent mouth tells stories about your heart, immune system, gut, vitamin lack, and much more. After the medical examination is done, one can still paint the town red again.

Remember that the physical examination only looks at about 1–25 percent of you. The rest of you remains hidden from your doctor and the machines. Only you can give the doctor access to the other 75–99 percent of you. (These figures are anecdotal.) The other 75–99 percent of you rarely gets onto the exam table. These parts are made up of

- your mental wellness or lack of it;
- the heart that pumps tears of pain or joy through your emotional system; and
- that thing that peeks at the world from behind your eyes—that thing of yours that is not the brain and not the mind, that part of you that you do not understand well and yet it knows you so well. That part of you is what I, as a doctor, cannot describe in terms of your biological make up.
- the people who crowd your space; they do not enter the consultation room but do contribute to your health and ill-health.
- the empty, or loaded pocket or purse.

## Medical Ethics

This is about doctors respecting (or disrespecting) you, your person, your secrets, their profession, and themselves. Sometimes we as docs fall short on this, and you need to know the basics. As defined by Richard Norman in the book *The Moral Philosophers: An Introduction to Ethics*(1983), by ethics we are trying to understand:

- about the nature of human values;
- how we ought to live our lives; and
- about the things that constitute right conduct.

How do doctors make the right choice when faced with a number of values that are of equal but competing importance?

Medical ethics has four major pillars that ought to protect you under all circumstances. The pillars (principles) are described here briefly:

1. Autonomy.

The principle of autonomy deals with the following issues:

- No doc has power over your body; you are in charge of how the doc handles your body, what goes into it, and what is drawn out of it. Your urine can only be tested for sugar with your consent. We cannot set to draw your blood without good explanation and without your consent.
- Your health records should be kept confidential. No info regarding your health or lack of health may be given to a third party without your consent.
- You have the right to consent (or refuse to consent) to a treatment modality after having received adequate info. This is called "informed consent" or "informed refusal" (according to medical ethics experts). Before you say yes or no, you ought to have been given enough info by the doc.
- You have the right to choose your doc.
- If your ailment is not life-threatening, the doc also has a right to choose not to see you.
- Trustworthiness and truthfulness are key elements of medical ethics. This should work well for you if your medical story is truthful. What the doc tells you will also most likely be truthful.

2. Above all, the doc should do you no harm.

This is the big stick that prevents doctors from doing any harm to you. Your healer can cause you harm during the interview, physical examination, diagnosis time, treatment, record keeping, and whenever he or she talks about you and medical problem. We cause you harm if we discuss your disease with other doctors not involved in your care. It is even a bigger harm (crime) if we discuss your disease with non-medical people. It is not only the physical harm that is bad but also emotional or psychological harm is as bad as, or even worse.

Before you partake (or refuse to partake) in any treatment, your healer ought to have informed you about the benefit and risks. Owning up to our mistakes maintains or restores the trust you put in us. Benefits of your treatment should always outweigh risks. You have the right to consent or refuse to the treatment as long as you have been given detailed info about risks and benefits.

## 3. Beneficence.

This is a big stick that pushes the doc to do good to you at all times. Continuing medical education is an example of what your doctors do for your own good. As doctors keep abreast with developments in medicine, they do it for your welfare and their own development. Being evaluated by peers help docs to help you better. The knowledge acquired helps them a bit but helps you the most.

Docs who know their limitations do you more good than bad.

## 4. Justice.

An example is distributive justice. Imagine a medical facility with a very ill senior citizen (over ninety years old) who needs a blood transfusion; his or her life depends on getting transfused with a unit of blood. In the same medical unit are five severely ill newborn babies whose lives depend on emergency blood transfusions. The medical facility has only one pint of emergency blood that could save the life of one senior citizen or the lives of five newborn babies—just that one pint of blood.

For once, we shall give you, the patient, the stethoscope for a day. Decide who gets the blood transfusion. You are not being forced to play God here—just being given a privilege to put the fancy tube around your neck. Would you save the senior citizen, or would you save the five newborn babies? You have just that one pint of blood. Go ahead—be the doc! That is the so-called ethical dilemma in medicine that your doc struggles with daily.

## Things to Avoid during the Consultation

Do not criticize the last doctor you visited. It won't score you any medical points, and it is a waste of your consultation minutes and dollar. Instead, tell the doctor about what was found, tests done, treatment given, and your response to the treatment. You may state what your expectations were during the previous consultations and whether or not they were met. This gives the current doctor a clue about what went wrong in the last consultation without you bad-mouthing the previous doctor.

When you talk ill of your previous doctor, it gets your doctor wondering what your story about him or her will be when you visit yet another doctor. He or she will spend more effort on what your story about him or her is going to be than getting a diagnosis and treatment plan for you. There will be very little effort and time spent on finding solutions to your medical problems.

Do not start by praising your new doctor at the beginning of a consultation. This eats into your consultation time and dollar, and you may set up your doctor for failure. The doc may then spend more effort on proving you right than on getting you well. The doc may develop performance anxiety.

Medical miracles are made when patients describe their symptoms in simple terms, lay terms. Indeed, your doctor is also a layperson when it comes to what is going on inside of you. So give the doctor a simple but detailed story. In describing previously confirmed medical diagnoses or procedures, you may use those technical words that were used to describe the tests done, the diagnoses made, and the treatments given. Here you will be talking about what has already been proven and documented. (Such a description belongs in the sections of this book called "Past Medical Problems," "Past Surgical Problems," and "Past Gynecological History.")

Some patients are not particular about the age, gender, and experience of the doc. For them, a good name is enough. A good name depends on the doc's excellence in the ABCs of medical knowledge or his or her XYZs of being human. If you are pretty lucky, your doctor will be a good medic and a good human being. Word of mouth would do you some good here. If, despite being assured by friends, your gut feeling still disagrees, just cancel that appointment. But in this case, the health dollar for the day is gone.

You are not likely to get a good consultation if you have escorted a family member or a friend to a doctor and then decide to get a "quickie consultation" without an appointment. You will still pay the full consultation dollar for that brief medical encounter but get very little health in return. In the same vein (or is it in the same artery?), do not allow a family member or friend who has escorted you to the doctor to steal your consultation time. This happens when the doctor probes your symptoms well and then gives you a satisfactory explanation. Your friend then hijacks your consultation: "Doc, I also have this niggling kidney pain." Should the doc start probing your friend's symptom, your dollar is gone. Make it clear to your escort that this is your medical show, not his or hers.

## The Mighty Phone or Digital Device

The doctor's contact details are usually of two types. One set is for the non-urgent medical problem (cold cases) that can wait for a month.

This includes the office telephone number, e-mail address, and other digital means of contacting the doc's office.

The other set of contact details is the doc's cell phone number. This is a contact detail that any patient may use if his or her health is on fire (true medical emergency): sudden onset of vomiting blood, family member collapsed and is unconscious, seizures, and so on. With these kinds of medical emergencies, the doc won't mind being woken up at 3:00 a.m. on a Sunday. But calling your doc at this time of the morning on Sunday to make an appointment for a longstanding back pain may tire your doc out. Or worse still, the doc may be reluctant to take your call on a day when you really need urgent medical attention. You do lose a dollar, your health, or even life in such a case. You should only cry wolf on a day that is there is one.

Just as you have the liberty to choose or drop a doc, doctors also have the liberty to discontinue professional relationship with nagging patients, especially those who cannot differentiate between a non-emergent problems and true medical emergencies. Docs may also shun patients who frequently bypass the reception and ask doc to schedule their appointments. Of course an emergency would be treated totally differently; that is why a doc is one of the few professionals who do not usually turn off the emergency phone number. If you are too busy for the doctor's receptionist, then let your receptionist schedule the appointments for you. Spare your doc the task of scheduling your appointment.

Frequently calling the doc after midnight for problems that you have had for months or years is a drain on the doc's mental resources. The medic is also human, and there will be other patients waiting for *your* doc the morning after the late-night phone calls. Imagine your doc receiving five such late-night calls from other non-urgent callers when you are the patient to be seen first thing the following day: the late-night, nonemergency phone calls would have drained your doc of all of his or her mental resources. Your doc will be irritable and a poor listener—your dollar gone. You may also cause the other patients to lose their dollar the following morning. These poor patients are likely to consult with a tired doc the following day. Their dollar is lost, all because of your late-night (nonemergency) phone calls.

In conclusion, there is a lot that goes on during a medical consultation that has nothing to do with the basic medical science and clinical skills that your doctor has studied in the university. The politics of medicine is about the fact that both you and your doc are human at the end of the consultation; neither is inferior or superior. Both you and your doc are experts who should respect each other. Both of you are two simple creatures of a very complex Creator. You and your doc sometimes make life very complex.

# Twelve

## Medically Induced Pain
## (Medical Tests)

This is one of the biggest sources of cost escalation in a medical consultation. Both you and your doc may work together to reduce the cost of your consultation. The "ouch" may be due to the needle prick or the hole created in your pocket.

We draw a lot of blood for diagnostic purposes in the process of medical care. This is a territory dominated by probes, cameras (scans), and tests on bodily fluids. The tests cost a dollar to you and the state.

If it is watery, doctors will take it and run with it to the lab. Look at urine as an example; it tells the doc many inside stories. It can reveal the health (or lack thereof) of your kidneys, blood, pancreas, and liver. If your urine is sweet, you may have the sugar disease, diabetes mellitus. Docs of yesteryear must have diagnosed diabetes by tasting the patient's urine; it is the disease of sweet urine. We are lucky these days; we use a medical dipstick to test the urine for sugar. Additionally, illicit substances can also be discovered in urine. Urine can also reveal an infection of the bladder and kidney or damage to your muscles. Your urine is also a storyteller.

Always ask your doctor the following:

- Will the test help change the treatment plan?
- Can the disease or illness be treated without doing the test?
- Does the test have any undesirable effects?
- Would you lose an arm and a leg while paying for the tests?

It is important to know these things. Some tests are done to protect your doctor from your lawyer. Such tests do not help you but may help your doctor survive litigation in case you let your lawyer loose on the doctor. So sometimes you pay for your doctor's peace of mind. If you give your doctor some reassurance that you are not the kind to call on a lawyer, then you get to do only the essential tests. But doctors fear all patients when it comes to litigation, so much so that many docs practice "defensive medicine" by ordering unnecessary and costly tests. You pay for the trend of other patients suing doctors. Dollar gone.

Ask your doctor about the benefits and risks of the tests. Always insist on knowing the value that doing the tests could add. You may find that you lose little by avoiding some medical tests. You may leave out unnecessary tests and let the doc document that. You save a dollar.

The best time for checking messages on your digital devices during a consultation is when it is time for drawing blood. Your doctor will not mind that you are busy on a social platform while drawing blood. The device is a good distraction. You would have thrown dollars if you did social media during medical storytelling time.

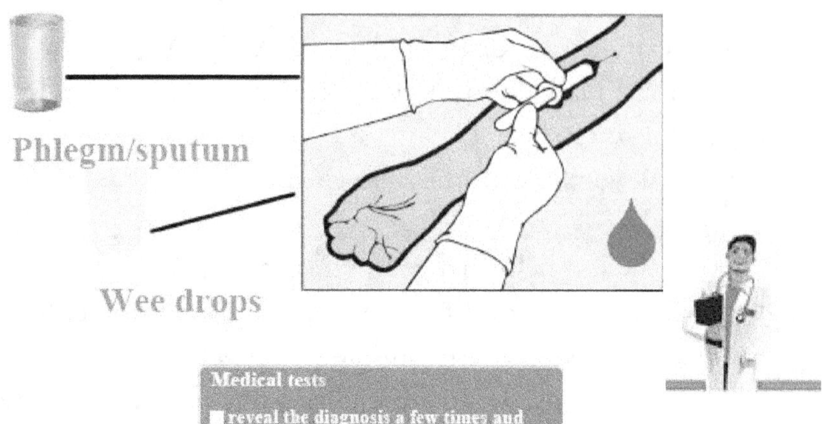
Phlegm/sputum
Wee drops
Medical tests
reveal the diagnosis a few times and
are fruitless and costly most times.

## The Pinhole Camera
## (X-rays and Scans)

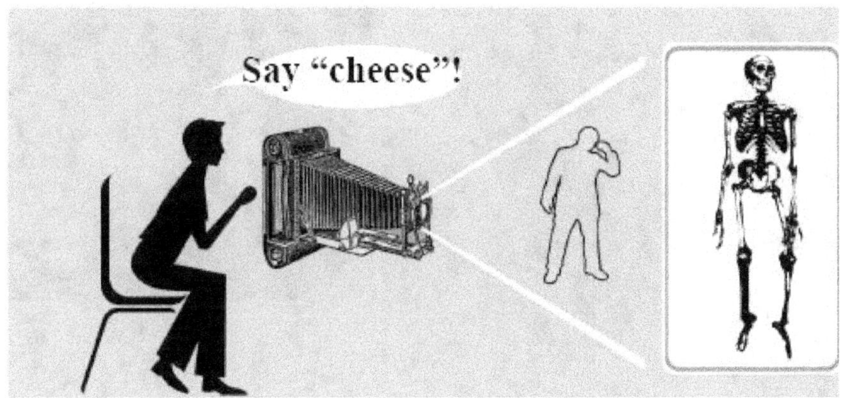



Ever wondered why the staff in x-ray departments wear protective clothing, hide behind thick walls before they take a "snap", and why they wear electronic tags every day at work? It is because their workplace puts them at high risk of developing cancers. They may soak up doses of radiation every day. Ever wondered why, if avoidable, pregnant women are not exposed to x-rays? We help the fetus avoid radiation. Of course, you are no longer in the womb and the dose you are exposed to is miniscule, but who wants to soak up multiple doses of x-rays over time? If not necessary do not take that pic.

If it is not really necessary, you and your doctor should make a habit of avoiding x-rays as much as possible. The more you get exposed to some scans, the more you are exposed to what the x-rays staff are protected from. You only get a tiny dose every shot, but if it is unnecessary why go for it? You also lose a dollar every time you get exposed to these rays.

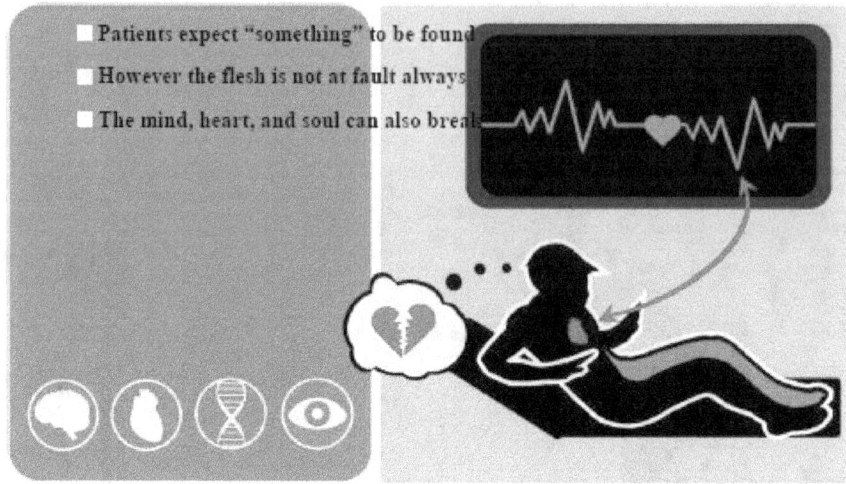


A *broken heart* may send the *medical heart* racing like a horse. That physical (medical) heart may race and be "sore," and yet the EKG/ECG and blood tests come out normal. When you have told your story well, the doc has examined you well, and the appropriate tests done, it can be clear which of the two hearts is indeed in need of therapy. The non-physical heart, even when "broken," does not require very costly medical tests—saving you a dollar at the end.

With any medical tests that have to be done, the level of discomfort or pain will be felt in your wallet and in your body. This is the *ouch factor* of medical tests.

# Thirteen



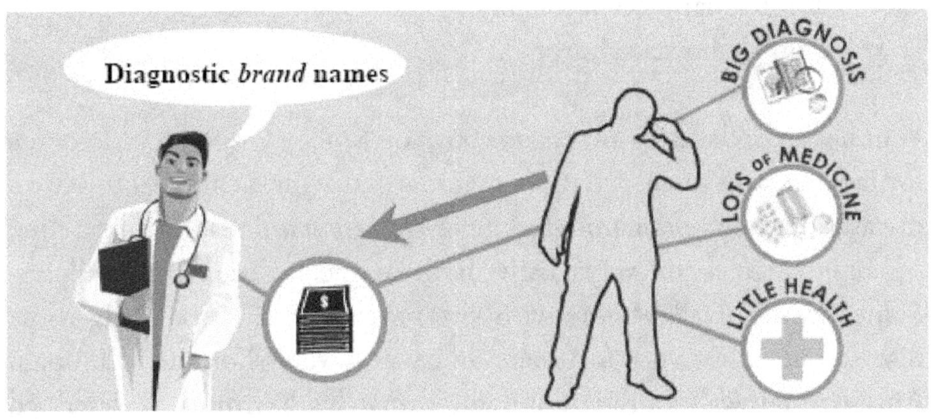


After the consultation, your near and dear ones want to know about it: "So what is the diagnosis? What did the doctor find?" They expect you to bring home a big diagnostic label, yet it happens on very few occasions.

Rarely does a patient go home with a fancy diagnostic label such as

- pneumonia of the right lung;
- chronic pancreatitis with mal-absorption syndrome; or
- chronic leaking ectopic pregnancy.

These sound great, but most medical consultations don't end up with such fancy diagnostic labels.

Most likely, you are going to walk home with some *unbranded* medical names like

- chronic low-back pain;
- adjustment disorder with anxiety;
- functional chest pain;
- chronic daily headache; or
- irritable bowel syndrome.

Your health dollar does always not buy you a fancy Greek or Latin name for tagging your disease. Believe me, it is better (and cheaper) to have a disease with no *brand* name than a big *brand-name* disease with no cure!

Brand names are very costly, both in the mall and in medicine. Someone who walks home with chronic pancreatitis has a big-name disease but is not very fortunate and will have a shortened life-span. Another may walk home disappointed that his heartburn is described by his doctor as non-ulcer heartburn, yet he has

- similar symptoms to the patient with pancreatitis;
- paid the same dollar for the consultation; and
- walked out without a fancy disease brand name and supplied with "air" only (a no-pill management for the no-name diagnosis).

The doctor whose patient walks out with non-ulcer heartburn is very excited that the patient did not have "chronic pancreatitis," while the patient is unhappy that he or she has not been given a diagnostic *super-name* to take to family and friends. The patient depicted below is a rare type; he is excited that his doc has given him a no-brand-name illness, which only requires lifestyle changes to sort out. He is excited that doc supplied him with air, no pills.

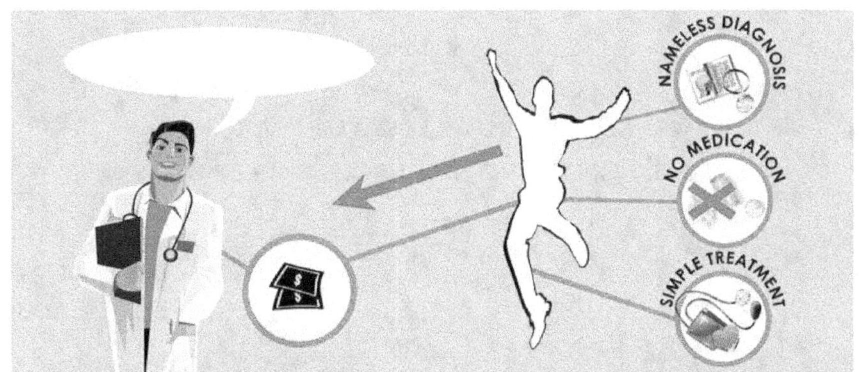


***The doc says nothing because there is no fancy medical word to utter. This is the so-called "no-brand-name" diagnsosis.***

As a doctor, I would be quite glad that the chest pain that sent me to consult with another doc is a functional chest pain (small-name diagnosis) and not angina pectoris (big-name diagnosis). Angina pectoris is a diagnosis that a doc does not want as a reason for his or her chest pain. It spells a shortened life-span.

The big-name diagnosis may sound great when you tell friends and family. It makes your doc sound great for coming up with the fancy name. Secondly, the *culprit* that caused you pain and suffering has a name and can be *crucified* by the doc. But lucky is the person who has a no-name diagnosis like *stress-related chest pain*, because he or she gets to live longer (and spend less) than the one whose chest pain is caused by an *acute coronary syndrome*. It is a good medical deal to go home with a no-name diagnosis plus a *bag of air*—no pill in hand, no side effects and a small coin spent.

# Fourteen

## Time for Air Supply
## (No Elixir, No Pills and Needles)

Treatment
("Management" is more politically correct word)

Every time we prescribe a pill, we legally give you a *poison* in nonlethal doses.

That small, nonlethal dose may be good for you but lethal for some other patient. Botox is one of the world's most potent poisons, yet it has plenty of medical uses. It is a wonder drug in Aesthetics, neurology and pain control.

Usually no body walks into a store with a dollar and comes out with nothing; often there is a grocery bag in hand, or a bill has been settled in store. When patients walk in for a medical consultation, there is normally that urge to walk out with *something* (a fancy medical diagnosis, medical tests, or a prescription.)

Treatment has this connotation that since you brought a dollar to the doc, you are expected to walk away with a pill. Management of a medical problem takes a different route. Treatment is a small part of management. In treatment your doc finds a disease, gives it a brand name, gives you pills, you down the pills, and the disease runs for its life.

When it comes to management of an illness, the rules change in the following ways:

- You and your doc draw up the list of your problems (with or without fancy medical names).
- You and your doc decide how many *bloody tests* you can stand or can afford.
- You and your doc have shared roles in fixing the list of problems, but you, being the generous and sick one, will take greater responsibility. You may excuse the doctor from doing physical exercise for you, because even if you paid the doc to help you, the disease is yours. On that note, you do the exercises, and the doc remains a couch potato (in respect of your disease). On a lighter note, I do exercise on behalf of some of my patients who pay me triple the normal fee. And indeed, they end up with surfboards for tummies without breaking a sweat! They also end up with good cardiovascular health because of the exercise that I, their doctor, do on their behalf. May be you should try this with your doc; I wonder whether it will work.
- The doc doesn't treat you; the two of you are managers of your list of medical and other problems. You manage the problem list together with you doing most of the work.
- You and your doc divide the problems into medical problems and nonmedical problems. If there is a need to walk frequently around the block, that is your pill.

I foresee an ideal patient in the near future who shall be very disappointed with a doctor who forces pills down his or her (patient's) throat.

Most family physicians know that a treatment plan is not to be forced down a patient's throat.

Currently many patients are still attracted to that kind of doc and run away from the doc who just supplies air, the infamous *no-pill* solutions.

Some medical problems will require a pill; others will not. When there is a need for a pill, you should let your doc take a break, and you pop the pill yourself. With all illnesses/symptoms, you should ask the doc if there are no-pill alternatives (air supply).

For the nonmedical list of problems, you and your doc will consider non-pill solutions, and again you give the doc a holiday. If you live in a burning house, you are not likely to ask the doc for a pill to stop the domestic fire. If you have to walk or jog your way back to health, give the doc a break and do the walking, jogging, dancing, or the swimming.

With management of a medical problem, sometimes less is more. You may be surprised that one medical problem can have up to thirteen symptoms. After giving the doctor your health dollar in exchange for a diagnosis and management plan, do not expect thirteen pills for the thirteen symptoms of a panic attack. You may be very surprised that all thirteen symptoms can be sorted out with just one pill—literally a pill for all the ills and not a pill for every ill, as they say. Sometimes air supply (talking therapy) may be all that you need for all those symptoms.

If the management plan is going to work, it has to be mutually discussed and agreed upon by you and your doctor. Usually you, as the patient, are given the working diagnosis or final diagnosis or the no-brand-name problem list. A working diagnosis (or the other likely diagnoses) gives you and the doc the possibilities of diseases/illnesses that are lurking inside you. We have a tentative disease label (the number-one suspect) to work with while searching for the final diagnostic label, which may be the same as the working diagnosis or totally different.

As an example, chest pain, pounding heart, sweatiness, tremors, breathlessness, and lack of sleep could be due to a panic disorder. This is the working diagnosis, but it does not mean that your doctor has discarded the idea of heart disease, thyroid disorder, or blood clots in your lungs. Medical tests or referrals will be based on the search for these other possible diagnoses.

## Hard Work with No Pay (Exercise)

If there is any pill with a long list of benefits and few side effects, it is physical exercise. Exercise is

- easily and readily available;
- affordable;
- accessible;
- underutilized and everybody has it in his or her drug cabinet;
- underrated by patients because it is cheap;
- only mentioned by doctors as a *by-the-way*; and
- accompanied by manageable, temporary, and minor side effects.

Many patients do not take this "pill" seriously, because it is too readily available and too simple. Worse still, it is free (and like most free things, it is not valued.) It is more commonly available than the legendary acetaminophen (paracetamol), and everyone knows about it. Exercise is also a safe, legal, and medically acceptable source of a natural high and painkiller (endorphins). Those who get addicted to the natural highs of exercise are difficult to "rehabilitate"; once hooked on exercise, they are unlikely to get off it. That is an "addiction" I wish upon all my patients.

Patients who religiously take this treatment eventually become less of patients and more of normal people. People who do not perform hard-work-without-pay regularly tend to become patients frequently in the long run. After many months, the pay-off for people who exercise regularly is big even if there is no paycheck (salary) at month end.

Patients who take this advice seriously take less and less dollar to the doc, but your doc will still insist that you get active and stay out of his or her consulting rooms. When you stay away from our medical suites, your dollar stays with you. When you frequent our rooms because of lack of "hard-work-with-no-pay," your dollar follows you to the consultation room. We try hard to keep you and your coin away from our rooms.

The number of symptoms and diseases controlled by exercise is reason for volumes of books. There is so much empirical research and so many anecdotal personal stories about the benefits of exercise. The less you use this pill, the more dollars doctors make out of you.

## Manipulating the Meal

The dietician/doc may call it a fancy name: dietary modifications, going on a diet, starvation trip, and so on. Manipulating the dish with your dietician/doc entails the following:

- Reducing, avoiding, or working on cravings.
- Allowing you to enjoy any meal, but much as some meals may be enjoyed four or five times a day (fruit and vegetables), others are best eaten only once a day, only once a week, and so on.
- Keeping a "don't touch" list to a minimum, especially where there are allergies, food intolerance, or organ failure.
- Avoiding the business of starving yourself, or denying yourself the goodies that God gave us; just remember the words "in moderation." A slice of cake a week won't make you obese, but seven slices a day for a month could give your doc big business. Moderation allows you to enjoy any dish (in moderation). If moderation were a meal, it would also to be enjoyed in "moderation."

## Manipulating Your Thoughts

Your doc may describe this with a tongue twister, cognitive behavioral therapy (CBT). This is done with or without the help of a therapist. This helps you to get your mind to listen to you, not the other way around. Most of us seek packs of pills to tell our minds to shut up. It is because our minds are in charge of us, and we follow haplessly. CBT allows your mind to listen to you. Do not get upset if the only pill you take home is CBT, because it is a very vital form of "air supply."

Thought manipulation is done by you with the help of those in the know, but you do the bulk of the work, subsequently avoiding a pill burden—a dollar saved. You get a big bang for your buck without downing a pill sometimes. Some psychiatrists put CBT at par with pills for management of some mental illnesses.

Even without spending a dollar, you can train your mind to mostly be where you are. Getting the mind to stay with the body is no easy task, but it is not impossible. Many of you bring us a dollar because you and your mind spend so much time away from each other; the infamous autopilot runs your lives while the mind is busy elsewhere, far from the flesh. Many self-help books and websites on meditation are available to help keep your mind on a short leash. Once your mind stays with you in everything that you do, you get health without spending a dollar.

## Manipulating Your Mouth

If negative things constantly come out of your mouth, then negative things are bound to go into your body. Some of these negative things will manifest in the form of ills that bring you and your dollar to us.

Let positive things come out of your mouth consistently, and your flesh will obey what the mouth spews out all the time. This also goes for what you put in the mouth and how frequently you do it. A change in this is a change in health, negative or positive, depending on what you put in or what you speak out. You can deny the doc a dollar or enrich the doc, depending on what you put in your mouth (and how frequently). To get well or stay well, some things need to approach your mouth more than three times a day. Other stuff may only get into your mouth once a day or once a week, and so on. Get the balance: do not starve, crave, or do a crash diet; and God will be glad that you have used (in moderation) everything yummy that he gave us.

## Manipulating Your Heart

Forget the blood pump, located in your chest, that moves blood around your body. We are talking about the other heart that doctors cannot see on an x-ray of your chest, the heart where you place happiness and sadness. That is the heart that your doctor cannot medicate, the nonmedical heart.

However big a truckload of pills your doc gives you, it won't change what you are responsible for placing into or removing from your heart. There are some basic things you are responsible for placing into or removing from your heart:

- Anger. Usually it is the duty of some "fool" to make you angry, but maintaining the anger is your duty; getting rid of it is also your job.
- Bitterness. Again, some other fool pours a dose of bitterness in your heart, but it is your job to keep it simmering inside or take it to the trash can.
- Cruelty. Whether you are the receiver or the supplier, cruelty causes and maintains some forms of illness.
- Deceit. Whether you are the supplier or the receiver of perpetual deception, you are bound to battle with some symptoms for a long time, despite a bucketful of pills.

- Envy. Practice this daily for a year, and see if what results is health or ill health.
- Fear that overwhelms faith. Get exposed to morbid fear regularly, and see what it gets you at the end of a year.

As you have seen, some illnesses will linger for a long time irrespective of adherence to medications, until some things change. The doc does not change these things for you; you do.

## Don't Try to Manipulate the Crowd

Trying to change the people around you (the crowd) to walk, talk, and dress like you will make you *dine* on pills for a long time. No doctor will sort your problem with pills if you don't like or do not fit into your crowd. Remember your crowd cannot fit into you; you have to fit into the crowd.

By the time your Creator was done creating the crowd around you, he was convinced that they were all created in his likeness. Trying to manipulate God's people will cause you social pain. Your doc won't have a pill for this illness. Changing yourself to fit into the crowd or fleeing the crowd may be the best option. When you escape from your usual crowd, hope that the next crowd will be exactly the way you want it, lest you try to change the new crowd as well. Good luck. Accept your crowd the way it is and save a dollar.

## Pills for Spiritual Pain

Your doc may give you a long prescription for this kind of pain, but the local pharmacies/chemists are not likely to have those medications in stock. This kind of pain (which also manifests as bodily pain) will require non-pill therapy; there is no pill for this ill. Air supply in mega doses would do a lot of good here. (Another book will deal with this in detail—coming out later.)

## Pills and Needles

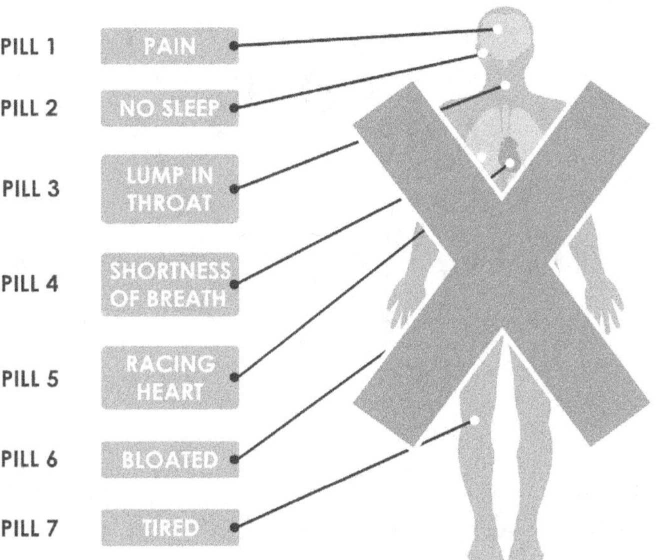


Taking a pill for every symptom will give you seven more reasons to see your doc again—seven sets of side effects from seven pills meant to treat seven symptoms! This is a nasty game of *seven-seven-seven* that you may not win.

Your doc may help you the most by giving you nothing physical but giving you loads of info, a major form of air supply. At least you will not go home with a pack of side effects in the form of medicines. A wise health-care provider of years gone by summed it up well: "All medicines are poisons, but poisons in small doses are the best medicines." Every pill that the doc prescribes for you is a poison but in an acceptable dose. You should take our "poisons" only when unavoidable.

The choice is entirely up to you: a big bang for your buck or a small bang for your buck. The buck is your health dollar, and the bang is the amount of health you get in exchange for that dollar.

# *Fifteen*

## *Avoid* Getting a Small Bang for Your Buck

*End of Consultation*

1. Question Time, Again

This time you become the interviewer; it is your turn to ask the doc questions. Please ask questions relating to the consultation, the blood tests and cameras (x-rays and scans), and the cost (an arm and two legs?)

Ask questions like the following:

"If the disease does not improve, when may I consult with you again?"

"Is it going to limit my life or affect the quality of my life adversely?"

"What changes do I need to make in order to speed up my recovery?"

"What do you mean by *dyspnea* and *key-hole surgery*, Doctor?" Do not assume that you are talking about the same thing, if uncertain ask the doc. Ask doc to clarify every "medical bomb" (medical jargon) he or she drops.

"Will I die?"

To this last question, your doc will reply, "Yes. Like the rest of us, you will also die—but may be not likely from that disease." And please know that death is not the problem; it is the fear of death and dying that is problematic (even for doctors).

Don't waste your consultation dollar asking about where your doc plays golf, though you two can discuss golf if your doc pushes the consultation toward that. You may ask virtually anything related to your health (flesh, heart, mind, your crowd, belief system, and the small voice inside you). Also, ask questions about your work and state of your wallet/purse if they bother you.

## 2. Safety Net

Usually, at the end of your consultation, you and your doctor hope that the best has been done, the final diagnosis has been made, and the correct management plan has been made. Sometimes this is not the case.

- Your doctor may have the wrong diagnosis.
- The diagnosis may be right, but the treatment may not be the right one.
- The right treatment might work in 90 percent of patients with the same diagnosis, but you might belong to the other 10 percent for whom the treatment does not work.
- The treatment may be the right one for the diagnosis, but you may be allergic to that specific medication.

Safety netting is the plan that you and your doc make about these possibilities. It is the plan B that you fall back on if your plan A does not work against the illness; plan B helps if plan A works against you.

This helps you and your doc plan for unseen eventualities, such as

- your symptoms not responding to the treatment plan;
- side effects of the treatment;
- new symptoms developing and getting out of hand; or
- your disease remaining rebellious despite a serious management plan.

## 3. Allocation of Duties and Commitment

Some patients are very frank and straightforward about what they are able or unable to perform:

- One patient may decide: "Doc, if these are the factors that caused my hypertension then I think I shall start working on them now. Let us leave the pills out for now and check after six months."
- Another would say: "doc I can see what the causes of my hypertension are, but currently I don't have the time; let us start with the pill and see what happens in six months." More dollars for the doc.
- A patient with an acute abdomen (surgical emergency) may opt to go home and think about the emergency surgery and get back to the doctor the next day. The doctor would not detain such a patient against his or her wish but records every detail discussed. This kind of patient is released with detailed info about the benefits and risks of his or her decision. If something happens to the patient at home, no one would (successfully) sue the doc. The patient's autonomy shall have prevailed over doc's wanting to do good, and the doctor shall have not caused any harm in this case. This is the *politics of medicine* at play.

The take-home message from this book can be summarized in less than a page. There is nothing wrong with heading to a medical consultation with your *medical shopping list* written down lest you forget the most important problem, or present the problems the wrong way around. You always write a grocery list, why not do it for your health? Your medical shopping list should have all the items that should get sorted:

- The main problem: a symptom or any problems of living. Expect your doc to give you time to elaborate on the main reason for consultation. The doc should ask more questions about this main problem, unless your elaboration was detailed.
- Other minor, but significant problems: these may be medical symptoms or any other problems of existence on planet Earth.
- Your past (or current, but controlled) medical problems: these are the known old medical/surgical/gynecological problems that may or may not be responsible for the new problems that have prompted you to consult today. Women who are pregnant should tell the doc.
- List of current or relevant past medications and other forms of therapy.
- Hobbies and habits that may or may not seem to be relevant to your reason for consulting.
- The job that you do, are looking for, or have lost. Your passion or hatred for your job should also make the list.
- Expect a relevant, decent, and appropriate physical medical examination.
- Expect some relevant but cost-effective medical tests.

- Time allowed for you to ask relevant questions, raise your fears, worries, concerns, hopes, expectations, and feelings about your medical shopping list.
- Expect to walk home with something, and sometimes that something may turn out to be nothing tangible. There may be no "pill for your ill."
- The treatment you receive should be ethical and given professionally. Your story should be truthful, and you should play your part in avoiding pills for every ill.
- Expect a safety net on which to land if your medical shopping list causes you harm or does not give you the desired outcome.

When the patient is child there may be significant differences in the story telling; the care-giver plays that role. Autonomy of the infant, toddler and young child is handed over to care-giver, or the state.

# Conclusion

With the knowledge gained from this book, you can always aim for a big bang for your buck—*avoiding a small bang* at all times. Just like you get the worth of almost every dollar you take to the grocer, ensure that you get the most out of your health dollar.

If you practice these skills daily during your medical consultations you avoid becoming one of those people who go on to develop chronic pain syndromes. Then luckily for you there will be no need to read the other books that will follow after this one; they will target those for whom Chronic Pain syndromes are already established and become problematic.

Anderson, E. D. C., I. W. Campbell, and J. A. A. Hunter. "General Examination and External Features of Disease." In *Macleod's Clinical Examination*. 10th ed., edited by John F Munro and Ian W Campbell. London: Churchill Livingstone, 2000. Chap 2; 23-70

Andersen, U. S. *Three Magic Words: The Key to Power, Peace and Plenty.* California: Melvin Powers, WILSHIRE BOOK COMPANY, 1954.

Blitz, J. "Communication Skills." In *Handbook of Family Medicine*, edited by Bob Mash. Cape Town: Oxford University Press, 2004.

Boon, Nicholas Al, Nicki R. Colledge, Brian R. Walker, and John A. A. Hunter, eds. *Davidson's Principles and Practice of Medicine*. 20th ed. Philadelphia: Churchill Livingstone Elsevier, 2006.

Bresick, G. "Family-Oriented Primary Care." In *Handbook of Family Medicine*, edited by Bob Mash. Cape Town: Oxford University Press, 2004.

Cassidy, Jim, Donald Bisset, Roy A. Spence, and Miranda Payne, eds. *Oxford Handbook of Oncology*. 3rd ed. New York: Oxford University Press, 2010.

De Villiers, M. "The Consultation—A Different Approach to the Patient." In *Handbook of Family Medicine*, edited by Bob Mash. Cape Town: Oxford University Press, 2004.

Kyabgon, T. *Karma: What It Is, What It Isn't, Why It Matters.* Boston. Shambhala, 2015.

Longmore, Murray, Ian B. Wilkinson, and Supraj Rajagopalan, eds. *Oxford Handbook of Clinical Medicine*. 6th ed. New York: Oxford University Press, 2004.

Mash, B., and J. Blitz-Lindique, eds. *South African Family Practice Manual*. 2nd ed. Pretoria: Van Schaik Publishers, 2006.

Masterton, G., and A. D. Toft. "The Principles of a Clinical Examination." In *Macleod's Clinical Examination*. 10th ed., edited by John F Munro and Ian W Campbell. Edinburgh: Churchill Livingstone, 2000.

McWhinney I. R. *A Textbook of Family Medicine*. New York: Oxford University Press, 1989.

Mfenyana, K. and B. Mash. "A Different Context of Care." In *Handbook of Family Medicine*, edited by Bob Mash. Cape Town: Oxford University Press, 2004.

Moodely, K. "Family Medicine Ethics." In *Handbook of Family Medicine*, edited by Bob Mash. Cape Town: Oxford University Press, 2004.

Norman, R. *The Moral Philosophers: An Introduction to Ethics*. Oxford: Clarendon Press, 1983.

Swash, M., and S. Mason. *Hutchinson's Clinical Methods*. 18th ed. East Sussex: ELBS Bailliere Tindal, 1984.

Taylor, R. B. *Manual of Family Practice*. 2nd ed. Philadelphia: Lippincott Williams & Wilkins, 2002.

Watson, M., C. Lucas, A. Hoy, and J. Wells. *Oxford Handbook of Palliative Care*. 2nd ed. New York: Oxford University Press, 2009.

Whittaker, D. "Illness, the Patient and Family." In *Handbook of Family Medicine*, edited by Bob Mash. Cape Town: Oxford University Press, 2004.